11/02

Adolescent Depression

A Johns Hopkins Press Health Book

FRANCIS MARK MONDIMORE, M.D.

Adolescent Depression

A Guide for Parents

The Johns Hopkins University Press

Baltimore & London

Note to the reader: This book is not meant to substitute for medical care of people with depression or other disorders, and treatment should not be based solely on its contents. Nor is it meant to offer legal advice, which must be obtained from a practicing attorney.

© 2002 Francis Mark Mondimore
All rights reserved. Published 2002
Printed in the United States of America on acid-free paper
9 8 7 6 5 4 3 2 1

The Johns Hopkins University Press
2715 North Charles Street
Baltimore, Maryland 21218-4363
www.press.jhu.edu

Library of Congress Cataloging-in-Publication Data

Mondimore, Francis Mark, 1953–
   Adolescent depression : a guide for parents / Francis Mark Mondimore.
       p.   cm. — (A Johns Hopkins Press health book)
Includes bibliographical references and index.
   ISBN 0-8018-7058-5 (hardcover : alk. paper) — ISBN 0-8018-7065-8 (pbk. : alk. paper)
   1. Depression in adolescence—Popular works. I. Title.   II. Series.
   RJ506.D4 M66 2002
   616.85′27′00835—dc21
2001007992

A catalog record for this book is available from the British Library.

Figures 3-1, 3-2, 3-3, 5-1, 5-2, 5-3, 7-1, 8-1, and 14-1 by Jacqueline Schaffer.

20 pbs

In loving memory of my parents,

Frank and Winifred Mondimore

Contents

Preface

For a long time, mental health professionals thought that serious depression was an illness only adults were likely to develop. The general belief among psychologists and psychiatrists was that children might get a little sad or upset about some disappointment or frustration but that they weren't emotionally mature enough to experience true depression. Gloominess and "angst" were thought to be almost universal among adolescents, but only temporary—just a developmental stage that they would emerge from unscathed.

Research done in the 1990s demolished these myths. We now realize that young people do indeed get seriously depressed. In fact, as is becoming clear, depressive illnesses and bipolar disorders that start in adolescence may be more serious and more difficult to treat than adult-onset mood disorders. A 1996 study sponsored by the National Institute of Mental Health estimated that more than 6 percent of young people between the ages of 9 and 18 years suffered from some depression during the six-month period of the study, almost 5 percent of them suffering from the serious depressive illness called major depressive disorder.[1] It's been estimated that nearly one in five persons will go through a period of serious depression during their lifetime, and research increasingly indicates that many of these people had their first encounter with depression as teenagers.

With the introduction of the new antidepressant medication Prozac (fluoxetine) in 1989, the treatment of depression entered a whole new era. Because the newer medications are so much safer and easier to take than the older ones, many more people started getting treatment for serious depression, and because so many more individuals were being successfully treated, serious depression became more widely recognized as a medical illness, as "medical" a problem as is diabetes or heart disease. This recognition has come about much more slowly for depression in young people, largely because of the myths about adolescent depression I mentioned earlier. Parents still struggle with the idea of their child being treated for a psychiatric illness, seeing a therapist, or taking medication for a problem that they may think—and hope—might, after all, be "just a phase." I hope to persuade you in this book that serious depression in adolescents is an illness—an illness that can be effectively treated.

Clinical studies have shown that depression is underdiagnosed in young people and undertreated as well. A study in 2000 found that only 20 percent of seriously depressed adolescents in a community sample received any treatment for their problem. The same study found high rates of relapse in these youngsters, and even more disturbing was the finding that, by their twenty-fourth birthday, many of them had developed other psychiatric problems in addition to depression, most especially alcoholism and drug abuse.[2]

We now know that depression comes in many forms and is often the symptom of a collection of emotional illnesses that psychiatrists call mood disorders. Some adolescents with a mood disorder are troubled by "down" and sad feelings—the feelings people usually think of when they hear the word *depression*. But other adolescents with a mood disorder have predominantly irritable moods with angry outbursts, temper tantrums, and destructive rages, problems that seem to bear little relationship to what most people think of as depression. Can the same illness really look so different in different young people? Why? These are some of the questions I hope to answer in this book.

This is not a "how to talk to your teenager" book. Adolescent mood disorders are complex, poorly understood, and potentially dangerous illnesses, and parents want the facts about these illnesses. What are the danger signals of serious depression in teenagers? How are mood disorders diagnosed? What are the implications of the different diagnoses? How does depression relate to other problems, like drug abuse, attention-deficit/hyperactivity disorder (ADHD), and eating disorders? What are the available treatments? How can parents of an adolescent with a mood disorder help their child get the best treatment possible? What else can parents do? You'll find answers to all these questions in this book.

I have organized the book into four parts. Part I, Symptoms, Syndromes, and Diagnosis, focuses on recognizing serious depression in adolescents and on understanding why mood disorders are real illnesses. It reviews some of the unique issues of emotional development during adolescence that may explain why mood disorders express themselves differently in young people than in adults. I also try to explain something about the diagnostic process in psychiatry and the classification of mood disorders.

Part II, Treatment, reviews the different medications and other medical treatments used to treat depression, as well as the different types of psychotherapy and counseling that have been shown to be useful, how these very different treatments relate to each other, and why a combination of both is the most useful approach to treating depression.

Part III, Variations, Causes, and Connections, discusses other problems that often complicate the picture in depressed adolescents, such problems as ADHD and eating disorders and the dangerous and frightening issues of suicidal behavior and "cutting." A chapter on the inheritance of mood disorders and evidence for the genetic basis of these illnesses rounds out this part of the book.

Part IV, Getting Better and Staying Well, contains the real-world, practical information you need to maximize the effectiveness of treatment and minimize the chances of relapse and complications. Finding a good treatment team, dealing with insurance issues, and handling such emergencies as dangerous behaviors and hospitalization are some of the issues covered here.

I hope that after reading this book you will better understand the symptoms, the treatments, the complications, and what we know about the causes of depression and bipolar disorders in adolescents. More importantly, I hope you will feel better equipped and more confident about helping your depressed adolescent get the most out of treatment, on the road to recovery, and on the path to becoming a happy and healthy adult.

Acknowledgments

I'd like to thank those who have helped me in the writing of this book. First, many, many thanks to Sallie Mink, R.N., of DRADA (Depression and Related Affective Disorders Association) at Johns Hopkins, who suggested the project to me in the first place and who was a constant source of support and encouragement.

Thanks to all my colleagues in the Affective Disorders Section of the Department of Psychiatry and Behavioral Sciences at Johns Hopkins, especially Anthony Drobnick, M.D., for feedback, encouragement, and support.

Thanks to Jacqueline Schaffer for her handsome illustrations, and special thanks to all the wonderful staff of the Johns Hopkins University Press, most especially my editor, Jacqueline Wehmueller. I have been fortunate indeed to work with such a dedicated and talented group of people.

And thanks, once again, to Jay Allen Rubin, my biggest fan and frankest critic, for always being there.

Introduction

For many years, psychiatrists and psychologists proposed that serious depression was rare, even impossible, in children and adolescents. We now know this is not true. In fact, you'll see the words *adolescent depression* in magazine articles and newspaper stories practically every day.

Often the term appears in a context that is very frightening for parents worried that their child may be depressed: a story about adolescent drug abuse or an incident of violence or, most terrifying of all, adolescent suicide. Parents can become so frightened at the thought of these destructive and violent problems affecting their family that they can't decide what to do next. Sometimes the thought "my child would *never* do something like *that*" tempts parents to minimize the severity of the symptoms of this treatable illness, perhaps allowing them to talk themselves out of seeking psychiatric evaluation for their teenager. On the other hand, it's possible to panic, perhaps rushing off to an emergency room in the middle of the night after finding some gloomy poetry that a teenager has left lying around. What should parents do if they think their adolescent might have a problem with serious depression? If an adolescent has been diagnosed with serious depression, what are the implications? How best to help?

I would be lying to you if I said that adolescent depression was something psychiatrists understand completely. But there is a lot we *do* know about depression in young people. Admittedly, quite a lot has been extrapolated from what we know about depression in adults, but nevertheless, we have enough facts to provide for a rational, logical approach to the diagnosis and management of this illness.

That word, *illness*, is key. What is unequivocally clear is that serious depression is the symptom of an illness—actually, a group of illnesses, called *mood disorders*. The symptom of depression should be approached in the same way *any* symptom that might indicate a serious illness is approached: taking the potential problem seriously, getting the adolescent to an evaluation by the proper professional expert as soon as possible, and participating in treatment by monitoring symptoms and treatment response, being supportive and encouraging, and participating in any other part of the treatment that the treatment team recommends.

The horror stories you read in newspapers are often the result of *not* following this approach: a serious depression that has gone unrecognized or, worse, that was suspected but not treated, for a variety of reasons: fear of a "mental illness" diagnosis, misinformation about psychiatric medications based on rumors and inaccuracies, or the erroneous idea that mood disorders are not "real" diseases. Parents of a child with diabetes don't generally worry over "what the neighbors will think" about their child's diagnosis and treatment. Parents of a child with leukemia don't usually blame themselves for their child's illness or wonder "what did we do wrong?" Serious depression *is* a serious medical illness and should be approached no differently from any other illness.

When the physician sees an adolescent who may be suffering from depression (I'll discuss later why a physician, specifically a psychiatrist, needs to be one of the first professionals involved), his or her approach will be the usual medical approach to symptoms and illnesses: getting all the facts about the symptoms, performing an examination of the patient, perhaps doing some lab tests, and making a diagnosis. The fact that symptoms are mostly emotional rather than physical ones—sadness, loss of interest in things, rather than abdominal pains or fever—doesn't change anything about needing a medical approach to what may turn out to be a medical problem. The examination involves talking and listening to the patient rather than using a stethoscope or blood pressure cuff, but psychiatrists have years of training that enable them, by just this method, to draw out mental experiences from patients and pick up subtle changes in psychological functioning that are the signs of illness.

Like physical illnesses, mood disorders have characteristic patterns of symptoms and a characteristic "natural history," that is, a predictable way in which the illness usually runs its course. To make predictions about a medical problem, first and foremost, a diagnosis must be made. The most important prediction a diagnosis allows is a prediction of what treatment will be effective at restoring the patient to health.

In psychiatric illnesses, as in no other group of medical problems, people get distracted by "why" questions and forget to focus on "what" questions. For the surgeon treating a person with a broken leg, *why* the patient's leg is broken (a car accident? skiing mishap?) is of relatively minor interest. The *what* question (What's wrong with this patient? His leg is broken *here* and *here*) is the focus of attention. The answers to these kinds of questions determine the treatment plan. Psychiatry is not that much different: treatment is determined by answering the question *what kind of depression does this person suffer from? Major depressive disorder?* The depression of *bipolar disorder?* The minor, temporary depression we call an *adjustment disorder?* The answer must be determined before other questions become relevant: is he depressed because he broke up with his girlfriend? Because he didn't get into the college that was his first choice? These kinds of questions are related to the search for diagnosis, but they usually become really relevant only *after* a diagnosis has been made.

This way of thinking about people and their emotions doesn't come naturally to us. We have all experienced being sad after a loss or apprehensive in the face of uncertainty, so we expect that all bad emotional feelings come about in this way. We have become accustomed to expecting to find reasons for unpleasant emotions in a person's life and experience. But this kind of analysis can lead us dangerously astray in the case of serious depression: looking for "reasons" can distract from the diagnosis, and thus delay the treatment, of a serious illness.

A more familiar example will illustrate. Perhaps your child, like many children, went through a period of having "tummy aches" on school mornings if she was nervous about school or simply didn't want to go. But the question "why doesn't my child want to go to school?" was probably *not* what popped into your mind that first morning, but rather: "*What's wrong with my child? What illness might explain these pains?*" It's probably a safe bet that you took the child's temperature, put her to bed and watched her closely, and perhaps called or even took the child to the pediatrician to make sure it wasn't an illness such as food poisoning or appendicitis that needed medical attention. You would wonder about the judgment of any parent who *didn't* take these steps, wouldn't you? Even a visit to the local emergency room wouldn't be an overreaction if the child seemed to be in extreme distress. Only *after* medical problems had been ruled out, when it was clear that the child wasn't ill, would it be appropriate to start looking for psychological explanations: reasons that the child might not want to go to school.

Parents are often the first to notice symptoms of depression, or perhaps just have a sense that something's not quite right with their adolescent, and just as the second grader with the morning tummy ache needed medical attention, the persistently sad or angry teenager does too.

The book begins, then, by describing the symptoms of these illnesses: mood disorders. Understanding how psychiatrists approach a problem with adolescent depression, make a diagnosis, and decide on a treatment plan is an important first step for the parent who wants know how to help.

PART I

Symptoms, Syndromes & Diagnosis

What is depression? Doesn't everybody feel "down" now and then, especially teenagers? How can we tell when depression is serious? These are some of the questions I'll answer in this first part of the book.

I begin with a chapter on what depression is, how to recognize it, and, more importantly, how it differs from the normal "downs" everyone experiences. This chapter also has an introduction to some of the theories of what causes depression, including a discussion of how we have learned that biological changes in the brain are at the root of serious depressive illness.

In chapter 2, I take a closer look at the psychology of adolescence and explain why depression often takes different forms in adolescents than in adults—so different that it may be hard to recognize.

Chapter 3 gets into the nitty-gritty of the diagnostic process in psychiatry, with an introduction to how psychiatrists think about depression and mood disorders, then an outline and description of the different types of depression that are seen in adolescents.

The part ends with a more detailed look at the diagnostic scheme for mood disorders that is currently used by the American Psychiatric Association: the *Diagnostic and Statistical Manual of Mental Disorders* (the DSM). I explain why it's important not to view the DSM as the "bible of psychiatry," as it often has been called, but rather to see it as an imperfect work in progress that is a helpful guide to, but not the ultimate authority on, the understanding and treatment of real-life patients in the real world.

CHAPTER I

Depression

Some Definitions

The word *depression* comes from Latin roots that mean "pressed down." Many of the common words we use to describe the feelings of depression describe, in one way or another, a downward direction or position. People talk about feeling "down in the dumps" or "low" or simply "down." The many synonyms for depression that begin with the same two letters, like "*de*spondent" and "*de*jected," share the Latin-derived prefix *de-*, which signifies a downward direction (as in "*de*scend").

Other words for depression cast it as the *opposite* of something: we say we are "unhappy" or "discontented," emphasizing the opposite of the good feelings of happiness or contentment. Still other words for depression conjure up the *absence* of something: the depressed are said to be "gloomy," a word that denotes an absence of light; or "dispirited," an absence of that vital spark of life we call spirit; or "desolate," the absence of just about everything. All these words capture something of the feeling of depression.

But if you listen to people who have suffered from serious depression talk about their experiences, you soon learn that depression is not a moving down or away from something and not really a lack of something; rather, it is a something that comes over its sufferers and imposes itself upon them. William James, the great nineteenth-century American psychologist-turned-philosopher, who suffered from depression, said that, far from an absence of something, depression is "positive and active anguish . . . wholly unknown to healthy life."[1] William Styron, the Pulitzer Prize–winning author of the novel *Sophie's Choice*, wrote in his memoir of severe depressive illness, *Darkness Visible*, of feeling "a poisonous fogbank roll in upon my mind."[2]

From the ancient Greeks comes the word *melancholy*, derived from their words for "black bile," the bodily fluid whose excess they believed caused the state of misery we now call depression. They conceptualized depression as caused by a disturbance of bodily functioning, an out-of-balance state of the four vital bodily fluids called "humors" (the other three were water, blood, and yellow bile). After several thousand years of attempts at other explanations, this idea should strike us today as an astonishingly modern one, an idea that some have now returned to with such phrases as "chemical imbalance" to describe where depression comes from.

But to define depression accurately, we need to define another word, *mood*, because any definition of depression must include the idea of *low mood*. Our mood includes our happiness or sadness, our state of optimism or pessimism, our feelings of contentedness or dissatisfaction with our situation, even physical feelings such as how fatigued or robust we feel. Mood is like our emotional temperature, a set of feelings that expresses our sense of emotional comfort or discomfort.

When people are in a good mood, they are confident and optimistic, relaxed and friendly, patient, interested, content. The word *happy* captures part of it, but good mood includes a lot more. The mental picture most people have of the boisterous adolescent is a good illustration of what *good mood* means. Teenagers feel confident and energetic and have a sense of physical well-being, they sleep soundly and eat heartily. It's easy for them to be sociable and affectionate; the future looks bright and the moment is ripe for starting new projects.

In a low mood, an opposite set of feelings takes over. People tend to turn inward and may seem preoccupied or distracted by their thoughts. The word *sad* captures some of the experience, but low mood is a bit more complicated. There may be a sense of emptiness and loss. People with low mood find it difficult to think about the future very much and, when they do, find it hard not to be pessimistic or even intimidated by it. Teenagers may be impatient and irritable, losing their temper more easily and then feeling guilty about having done so. They have difficulty being affectionate or sociable, so they avoid others and prefer to be alone. Energy is low, motivation ebbs away, and interest is dulled. Self-doubt takes over; they become preoccupied, worrying even more than usual about how other people see them. As you will see later in this part of the book, depression is sometimes complicated and difficult to spot, especially in adolescents. But the core feature of depression, its defining characteristic, is *low mood*.

NORMAL AND ABNORMAL MOODS

Some of life's more common stresses and the normal human reactions to them are such everyday experiences that common terms have been coined for some mood changes—and most people recognize these mood changes as quite normal. Moving to a new community where we don't know anyone often leads to a sense of dislocation and loneliness that we know as homesickness, an unpleasant experience that may last for days or even weeks, a mood that everyone has probably experienced at one time or another. When someone close to us dies, we experience a profound sense of sadness and loss that can become temporarily incapacitating—the deep sorrow that we call bereavement or mourning.

At the time of various milestones of personal achievement, we experience changes of mood in the other direction. On the occasion of a graduation or winning an important championship game or a coveted scholarship, a teenager can be filled with joy and pride and a sense of limitless optimism, feelings that can be nearly overwhelming. We wouldn't call any of these moods "abnormal," even though they can be extreme.

Like many other things we can measure in human beings—body temperature, blood pressure, hormone levels, for example—a person's mood state normally varies within a certain range. People, especially adolescents, are not in the same mood state for long; it is quite normal for everyone to have ups and downs of mood. So, low mood is sometimes *normal*. But there are other times when it is not, when it is the symptom of a *mood disorder*.

THE *SYMPTOM* OF DEPRESSION

Just like physical pain, then, periods of low mood are universal human experiences. People grieve when a loved one dies, are disappointed when an eagerly anticipated trip must be canceled, heartbroken when a romance ends unexpectedly. In these cases, feelings of depression seem normal. No one would think of low mood in such circumstances as a symptom of anything.

It's not difficult to think of situations when even physical pain can be regarded as almost normal. If the initial lawn mowing in the spring is the first bout of vigorous physical exercise after months of wintry inactivity, waking up the next morning with stiff and sore muscles is no surprise. Spend too much time out in the sun without proper protection and a painful sunburn results. But no one thinks of after-exercise soreness as a muscle disease or would call sunburn a skin disease. Some healing needs to take place in both cases, but neither makes one worry that something in the body isn't working as it should.

But if you woke up one morning after mowing the lawn with achy muscles and joints, *and* a fever, headache, and scratchy throat and cough, you wouldn't blame it on unaccustomed exercise. The other symptoms that accompany the sore muscles, especially the fever, indicate that something else is going on—in this case, probably a nasty virus. The *collection* of symptoms points towards a viral infection, even though one of the symptoms— the muscle aches—might be expected after too much physical exertion. A *clinical syndrome* includes a collection of symptoms and clinical findings that point towards a particular illness or group of illnesses.

When depressed mood is accompanied by certain other symptoms, such as disordered sleep and appetite, and includes severe irritability or a severe loss of energy and interest in usual activities, one should suspect that the individual might be suffering from a depressive *illness*—even if there are reasons that would explain one of the symptoms: low mood. Psychiatrists begin to consider the diagnosis of a mood disorder when they find that the patient has the *syndrome* of depression.

THE *SYNDROME* OF DEPRESSION

The core *symptom* of depression, low mood, can show up in many different situations, some of which can be called normal, such as feelings of bereavement during a period of mourning. The *syndrome* of depression indicates the presence of a serious medical problem that requires treatment. A case history will illustrate.

▼
───────────────────────────────

Susan had been thinking for weeks about how to bring it up to her husband. "Tom, I think we made a mistake taking Charlie out of Springfield."

"What do you mean?" said her husband, putting down the newspaper he'd been reading. "Edgemont is the best prep school in Columbia; how could it be a mistake? What makes you think that?"

Susan had closed her book and laid it on her lap. She looked down at its cover, then up at her husband sitting across the den, and said, "I think Charlie's unhappy at Edgemont. He misses his friends at Springfield."

Tom's face, which had frowned with concern briefly, relaxed at this. He picked up the newspaper from his lap and started to scan the columns again. "Is that all you're worried about? He'll get over it, Sue. He had to change schools twice during junior high because of our transfers and he handled it without any problems." Then, Tom lowered the paper again. "Does he talk about missing his friends?"

"Well, I asked him how school was going the other day and he told me he wasn't sure. He said he felt like he wasn't fitting in, that he's felt disconnected since school started."

"That's not so unusual for a kid starting at a new school at this age. Teenagers are so sensitive about that kind of thing."

"Charlie also said he's worried he might not be as smart as the kids at Edgemont. Tom, that's not like Charlie at all. He's a smart boy and he's always known it. He's always been so confidant about himself."

"Well, I still think it's some kind of adolescent phase. This is only November, Sue; give the kid a chance to settle in. Besides, it's not like he was against transferring into Edgemont."

Tom had gotten an important promotion within his company the previous spring—with a hefty salary increase. Tom and Susan could now afford to send their son to a prestigious private school and had asked Charlie what he thought about transferring. "Wow, that would be super!" Charlie had said enthusiastically. "Springfield is a good school and all, but Edgemont Prep! Have you seen their computer labs?"

Tom continued, "Charlie talked all summer about how much he wanted to join some of the computer clubs at Edgemont."

"Well, that's just it, Tom. He hasn't."

Tom's face became more serious. "He hasn't?"

"No. He seems to have lost interest in computers altogether."

"Are you sure?"

"Do you remember that computer graphics thing he ordered last month for his PC? So his computer games would work better? It finally came last week and I put it on his desk in his room." Susan looked down at her closed book again.

"I was putting clean clothes in his bureau this morning and I found it in the bottom drawer."

"Well, maybe it was the wrong piece; maybe it was incompatible or something."

"Tom, he hadn't even opened the package. He'd just stuffed it in a drawer."

"Wow, that's not like Charlie at all."

"Another thing," Susan continued. "He goes right to his room when he comes home from school and sleeps. I can't get him to come to dinner at all. I'm sure he's lost weight."

"Well, that's not so unusual, is it? Kids sleep more at this age, don't they?" Tom asked.

"I don't know—not this much, I don't think," said Susan. "Last Sunday, he was in bed most of the day *and* all night. That can't be normal."

"He has been extra quiet the past few weeks. Let me talk to him and see what I can find out."

"Please do, Tom. I'm worried."

Let's review the facts of this "case" for a moment. The most important fact is that Charlie's mother has noticed that Charlie is just not himself. Though you won't find this listed in diagnostic manuals, it's an important fact and typical of mood disorders. The individual seems to undergo a change in so many aspects of emotional life that those around him, even if they can't quite list details, notice that he is simply different. Sometimes parents have trouble pinning it down, but often, if they think about it, they realize that the activities, enthusiasms, and energy they've come to take for granted in their teenager seem to have drained out of him. Sometimes parents will be tempted to doubt these subtle intuitions that something is wrong and, like Tom in this vignette, ascribe what they notice to "a phase" their teenager is going through. This is usually a mistake. Susan has noticed that her son's energy level, motivation, and interest level have changed. Her intuition that this isn't normal is quite correct.

Psychiatrists use the word *anhedonia* to designate a loss in one's ability to enjoy things. It is one of the defining features of the depressive syndrome and worth discussing in more detail. Derived from the Greek work for "pleasure," *anhedonia* can be defined as loss of the ability to experience pleasure. One of Charlie's favorite things seems to be his computer—which makes his stuffing a new, unopened piece of hardware into a drawer an indicator of something very wrong. When depressed, adolescents will lose in-

Table 1-1 Symptoms of Depression

Mood Symptoms
   Depressed mood
   Pervasive, constricted quality of mood
   Irritability
   Loss of ability to experience pleasure (anhedonia)
   Guilty feelings
   Loss of interest in usual activities
   Social withdrawal
   Suicidal thoughts

Cognitive (Thinking) Symptoms
   Poor concentration
   Poor memory
   Indecision
   Slowed thinking
   Loss of motivation

Bodily Symptoms
   Sleep disturbance
      Insomnia
      Hypersomnia
   Appetite disturbance
      Weight loss
      Weight gain
   Fatigue
   Headaches
   Constipation
   Worsening of painful conditions

terest in sports, friends and socializing, extracurricular activities, or favorite classes or subjects. They are unable to derive any pleasure from listening to music, going to a movie, engaging in the sports or hobbies they usually enjoy.

Great writers, artists, and musicians who suffered from depression have left us poignant and vivid descriptions of this unresponsiveness to pleasure. In his novel *The Sorrows of Young Werther,* Johann Wolfgang von Goethe has his main character express a loss of responsiveness to the joys and beauty of nature: "Nature lies before me as immobile as on a little lacquered painting, and all this beauty cannot pump one drop of happiness from my heart to my brain."[3] People with depression describe food losing its taste, colors draining away from sunrises and landscapes, flowers losing their textures and perfumes—everything becoming bland, dull, and lifeless. For some, the bright and beautiful things in the world become a source of anguish rather than pleasure. The nineteenth-century Austrian composer Hugo Wolf described a terrible sense of sorrowful isolation during his depressions, a feeling of separation from the world of ordinary pleasures—all the more painful when it occurred in springtime:

> What I suffer from . . . I am quite unable to describe. This wonderful spring with its secret life and movement troubles me unspeakably. These eternal blue skies, lasting for weeks, this continuous sprouting and budding in nature, these coaxing breezes impregnated with spring sunlight and fragrance of flowers . . . make me frantic. Everywhere this bewildering urge for life, fruitfulness, creation—and only I . . . may not take part in this festival of resurrection, at any rate not except as a spectator with grief and envy.[4]

Now imagine what it is like when these terrible feelings come over young persons who are just learning to make sense of their feelings, adolescents who are still trying to understand their emotional reactions to the world. Young adolescents, especially, will have difficulty identifying and describing their internal emotional states, and the word *depression* often doesn't mean very much to them. This may be one of the reasons that low mood in adolescents sometimes is associated with prominent irritability. Frightened and frustrated by their depressive feelings, young people sometimes lash out at anyone and anything around them. In some adolescents, the irritability can even be the most prominent aspect of their change of mood.

Another differentiating factor between a "normal" low mood and the depressive syndrome is that individuals with a mood disorder lose the normal *reactivity* of their mood states. When persons who do not suffer from a mood disorder go through a period of low mood, such as after a romantic disappointment, the loss of a job, or a period of homesickness, they retain the normal *reactivity* of mood, that is, the normal changeability of mood in relation to what is going on around them.

Anyone who has attended a funeral and then returned to the home of the bereaved afterwards has probably observed—and perhaps experienced—this normal reactivity of mood. Mourners who might be grief-stricken during the funeral service or at the graveside can often relax, reminisce about good times they had with the person who has died, and enjoy catching up with friends and relatives perhaps not seen for a long time. The reactivity of mood is also retained in the lonely or homesick person who goes to the movies, can lose himself in a good film, and forget about his longing for more familiar surroundings. If the depressed mood is a "normal" one, we are able to dispel the feelings of bereavement, isolation, or disappointment—even if it's only for a few hours.

The depressed mood of the syndrome of depression, on the other hand, is *constricted*. Years ago, AM radio stations used to give away free radios, gifts that came with only one catch: they couldn't be tuned to any of the sponsoring station's competitors. These radios were built to receive only the signal of the station that gave them away. The mood state of the person suffering from a depressive disorder is like one of those radios, "set" to receive only one mood signal: depression. The mood of the syndrome of depression is a relentless, pervasive gloom that continues from one day to the next, week after week. As William Styron said of his own depression, "The weather of depression is unmodulated, its light a brownout."[5]

Another aspect of the depressive syndrome is a preoccupation with negative thoughts: depressed individuals often find their thinking dominated by thoughts of inadequacy or loss, regret, and even hopelessness. In depressed adolescents, worries about not "measuring up" in some way that seems out of character for them are not uncommon. Charlie's worry that he's not smart enough to compete in his new school would be a typical kind of negative thought, especially indicative of depression, since, as his mother says, he's never been troubled by such a worry previously. Guilty ruminations are especially characteristic of the syndrome of depression, and psychiatrists often make a special point to ask about guilty feelings when examining a person being evaluated for depression. Ruminations on themes of guilt, shame, and regret are common in the depressed states of the mood disorders, and they are uncommon in "normal" low mood states. An adolescent who talks about being responsible for his difficulties in some way, who describes himself as "lazy" or "worthless," is probably seriously depressed. Individuals experiencing the normal depressed mood that comes after a personal loss usually attribute their bad feelings to the fact that a loss has occurred—only in unusual circumstances will they think they are to blame for the problem and be preoccupied by guilty feelings or feelings of shame. The individual with a depressive syndrome, on the other hand, frequently feels to blame for his troubles, and sometimes for other peoples' troubles as well. The presence of guilty preoccupations is very significant for making a diagnosis of the syndrome of depression.

ASSOCIATED SYMPTOMS OF DEPRESSION

So far I've concentrated on the mood changes seen in the depressive syndrome. But there are other symptoms as well, changes beyond the change in mood.

Severe depression almost always causes a change in sleeping pattern. Depressed persons frequently suffer from insomnia—but also from its opposite, sleeping too much (*hypersomnia* is the technical term). A peculiar rhythmic pattern of sleep disturbance and mood changes through the day sometimes seen in depressed persons is called *diurnal variation of mood* (*diurnal* is a word used in biology to refer to a twenty-four-hour cycle). Persons with this pattern fall asleep at the usual time and without much difficulty but wake up very early in the morning after only a few hours of sleep. Lying awake hours before sunrise, they experience their lowest mood of the day during this early morning period, and minor problems and regrets seem magnified and overwhelming. They notice a gradual lifting of their mood as sunrise approaches, and when the morning light comes they can often rouse themselves and start their daily activities. As the day goes on, their mood continues to improve little by little until, by day's end, they feel nearly back to normal. They go to bed and can often fall asleep normally, but several hours later they awaken depressed, and the cycle repeats itself.

Appetite is usually disturbed in depressed individuals. As with sleep problems, changes occur in both directions: eating too much or too little. Individuals can lose or gain a significant amount of weight during periods of depression. (I discuss the deliberate self-starvation and compulsive eating of *eating disorders* in chapter 12; these behaviors seem to be complex syndromes of their own, perhaps a kind of complication of a mood disorder.)

Of the other bodily symptoms that occur in depression, a sense of fatigue with prominent low energy and listlessness is one of the most striking. Headaches, constipation, and a feeling of heaviness in the chest are common, as are other, more difficult to describe uncomfortable physical sensations. Whether these symptoms are caused by depression itself or arise from the lack of restful sleep, lack of exercise, and poor eating habits that depression brings is not clear. Depression seems to lower the pain threshold: depressed individuals seem more sensitive to pain and are more distressed by it.

Even young children can identify a physical pain and are able to describe a headache or stomachache, but they may not be able to identify and name a painful psychological state. The young adolescent who may not quite understand the concept of low mood may instead complain of headaches that make her want to spend time in bed. In young adolescents who are depressed, uncomfortable physical symptoms may result in frequent physical complaints that predominate over complaints of low mood.

Depression changes thinking as well as mood. Depressed persons can experience slowing and inefficiency in their thinking and often complain of memory and concentration problems. Charlie's complaint that he's not as smart as the other students in his new school might be understood better in this way. It's very possible that he is indeed not performing as well as some of the other students in his classes, but his concentration is probably adversely affected by his depression. When concentration is impaired, memory can seem to be affected as well: when we can't concentrate, our ability to register and later retrieve information is also impaired. Falling grades at school are very common in adolescent depression, and while certainly due in part to the energy and motivation problems depression causes, they are probably also caused by what psychiatrists call *cognitive* symptoms. From the Latin *cognoscere*, meaning "to know," this term refers to problems in concentration, thinking, and memory. We know, for example, that in depressed elderly persons, these sorts of thinking problems can be so severe that depression can be misdiagnosed as Alzheimer's disease.

MOOD DISORDERS: REAL ILLNESSES

Because everyone has gone through periods of low mood at one time or another, many people think they understand depression. Even the associated symptoms of the depressive syndrome sometimes accompany normal low mood states briefly or in a much milder form: a bit of trouble falling asleep for a night or two or a temporary loss of appetite are not that unusual after a serious disappointment or loss.

These facts can make it tempting to think that serious depressive disorders must follow the same "rules" as ordinary low mood states. They don't. Serious depressions don't get better on their own after a few days. Seriously depressed adolescents can't "shake off" their mood states or get their minds off their troubles by concentrating on school or sports or friends. They can't "get over" whatever preoccupations with loss or failure their depressive illness inflicts on them. They can't "get hold" of themselves or "shape up," "move on," "lighten up," do something about making some changes, or pull themselves up by their bootstraps—or any of the things people can usually do to get past a period of low mood. Adolescents with mood disorders are in the grip of their illness, and their symptoms stay with them day after day, week after week, relentlessly. It's thought that this is due to very real changes of functioning in certain brain "centers" or "circuits."

It is tempting, however, to fall back on our own experiences with low mood as well as our experiences with people in general and to attribute the seriously depressed adolescent's inability to "get over" her depression symptoms to being unmotivated, lazy or stubborn, or simply not trying hard enough. This misunderstanding of what serious depression really is can lead to very serious problems. At worst, it can lead to the conclusion that there is nothing wrong with the teenager that time or encouragement or stricter discipline won't solve. It might lead to the conclusion that the seriously depressed adolescent is simply "troubled" and that a few counseling sessions or a few weeks of talking to a therapist will take care of the problem. While counseling and therapy are certainly important aspects of the treatment of all types of depression, medical intervention, *treatment with medication*, is the mainstay of treatment of serious depressive disorder.

How do we know this?

THE CHEMISTRY OF MOOD

One of the greatest revolutions in medicine occurred during the seventeenth and eighteenth centuries, when physicians began to realize that the workings of the human body followed the rules of science. Indeed, the word *science* came to be used in its modern sense during this time and replaced the older term *natural philosophy*. Today, we take for granted that the heart is a pump and that we can understand a lot about the way it works if we understand how pumps work. After the Frenchman Pouseille elucidated the laws of physics that determine the flow rate, pressure, and other properties of liquids flowing through glass tubes, it quickly became apparent that the flow of blood through arteries and veins follows the same principles. "Philosophical" speculations on the heart as the source of love, loyalty, and other poetic qualities and feelings disappeared and were replaced by cold hard mathematical rules and principles.

It took several hundred more years for us to realize it, but, as is now quite clear, the functioning of the brain follows scientific principles as well and depends on processes that follow the rules of biochemistry (the chemistry of living things). We also know that the brain is the organ of emotions and thinking, so it follows that, at some level, thinking and emotions depend on these biological and chemical processes. It also follows that when those processes go awry, abnormalities of thinking and emotions result.

If you think about it for a moment, you'll realize that it really isn't such a new idea. People have used various chemicals to change thinking, emotions, and behavior for thousands of years. Almost as soon as we figured out how to raise crops, we discovered how to ferment some of them and began using ethyl alcohol (the alcohol in alcoholic beverages) to change the way we feel. We found substances that dull the perception of pain (aspirin from the bark of willows, morphine from poppies), substances that boost mood and energy level (caffeine from coffee beans, cocaine from coca leaves), and even substances that induce abnormal mental experiences such as hallucinations (*Psilocybe* mushrooms and the peyote cactus, among others). Ancient peoples attributed these effects to spirits or demons or gods, but during the early part of the twentieth century biochemists isolated the active ingredients from these natural materials, and several decades later neuroscientists discovered specific mechanisms of action for some of them (such as the discovery of receptors in the brain to which morphine binds). The number of naturally occurring psychoactive substances (those having an effect on the activities of the brain and nervous system) has now been far surpassed by the number of manufactured ones. We take it for granted now that chemicals, either naturally occurring or synthetic, can alter the biochemical functioning of the brain and thus alter thinking and emotions.

During the middle decades of the twentieth century, researchers discovered that several pharmaceuticals had very specific effects on *mood*. Reserpine is a pharmaceutical extracted from the root of an Indian shrub, *Rauwolfia serpentina*. Ancient Hindu writings mention the use of the plant for medicinal purposes, but not until the 1950s was it discovered to have a potent effect on blood pressure, becoming the first effective agent to treat hypertension (high blood pressure). As was also noted, some patients who took the medication to control their blood pressure developed serious depression. Low mood gradually developed over a period of weeks and soon was accompanied by all the other manifestations of the depressive syndrome—several patients taking this drug committed suicide.

In 1951, several doctors prescribing iproniazid, a pharmaceutical used to treat tuberculosis, noticed an interesting side effect in some of their TB patients: it helped with depression. Patients with low mood, sleep and appetite disturbances, and other symptoms of serious depression had a remission of these symptoms after taking iproniazid for several weeks. The first *antidepressant* medication had been accidentally discovered.

In part II of the book, in the discussions of treatments, you will see that *all* of the medications used to treat mood disorders were discovered more or less accidentally. But accidental or not, the discovery of pharmaceuticals that can cause the depressive syndrome and others that can make it better unequivocally points to the existence of a *biochemistry of mood*. A mood disorder, then, must be what occurs if something goes wrong with this chemistry.

In this chapter, I've started to give you a picture of adolescent depression, with an emphasis on the most common symptoms and an overview of some approaches to understanding it. In the next chapter, I fill in some details of this complicated picture with some facts derived from research on what is still a poorly understood illness.

CHAPTER 2

Normal Adolescence and Depression in Adolescence

It is not too far off the mark to say that our understanding of serious depressive illnesses in young people is several decades behind our understanding of depressive illnesses in adults. Fortunately, the field is catching up fast. But experts still disagree on many of the most basic facts about depression in adolescence. How frequently does serious depression occur in young people? What exactly are the symptoms? What is the best treatment approach? What are the risk factors for depression in young people? Are there protective factors? How likely is it that depression will continue to be a problem into adulthood for any given individual? Are there common complications of the illness?

MORE ON SYMPTOMS

Until the 1970s, depression in young people was thought to be "masked" or expressed in "depressive equivalents" rather than as a depressive syndrome like that seen in adults. Periods of depressive crisis during adolescence were thought inevitable and, even when extreme, were thought to be caused by extreme stresses or maturational problems brought on by pathological parenting or environments. Soon, however, research began to throw doubt on these ideas, and some facts about adolescent depression emerged. Adolescents (and children as well) show the same symptoms of depression as do adults and can develop the full depressive syndrome. In 1987, a study was conducted of 296 children and adolescents between the ages of 6 and 18 years who had been referred to a clinic specializing in child and adolescent depression and were carefully examined for depressive symptoms. A statistical analysis of the pattern of symptoms found that "the similarities across the school age in the [symptoms] of major depressive disorder far outweigh the few differences."[1] The clusters of symptoms included mood symptoms, negative thinking, anxiety symptoms, and appetite problems and paralleled the adult symptom pattern in both the children and the adolescents examined. A more recent study, focused on older adolescents (age 14 to 18), also found that depressed youngsters had symptoms typical of adult depression (see table 2-1).

This research also indicates that despite the similarities across age groups, some subtle patterns of symptom differences show up as one looks closely at different ages. Younger adolescents, like small children, seem to have more in the way of anxiety symptoms: fearfulness and nervousness. They show clinging behaviors, unexplained fears, and physical symptoms of anxiety such as stomachaches and stress headaches. Older adolescents suffer more from loss of interest and pleasure, and they have more in the way of morbid thinking: thoughts of death and suicide.

Another set of symptoms now recognized to occur in some severely depressed adolescents are what are called *psychotic symptoms*. *Psychosis* is an unfortunately vague term that is nevertheless frequently used in psychology to describe various symptoms of loss of touch with reality: specifically, hallucinations and delusions. Hallucinations are sensory perceptions without actual sensory stimuli: hearing voices when no one is present, seeing things that no one else can see. Delusions are false beliefs that preoccupy the person with such conviction that he cannot be persuaded otherwise. He may be convinced that he has a terrible incurable illness such as cancer or AIDS or believe his family has lost all its money, so that he will become homeless or institutionalized. In depressive illnesses, the delusional beliefs usually have depressing themes such as these, and the person may believe he has committed some terrible sin or crime and fear severe punishment. The hallucinations seen in psychotic depression are depressing as well: the individual may hear voices calling him bad names or condemning him, telling him he is worthless or a failure. The visual hallucinations are usually frightening and grotesque: of devils or monsters. Research has shown that hallucinations are more common in children than in adoles-

Table 2-1 Symptoms of Adolescent Depression

Symptom	Percentage of Adolescents Reporting
Depressed mood	97.7%
Sleep disturbance	88.6
Thinking difficulties	81.8
Weight/appetite disturbance	79.5
Anhedonia	77.3
Worthlessness/guilt	70.5
Loss of energy	68.2
Thoughts of death/suicide	54.5

Source: Peter Lewinsohn, Paul Rohde, and John Seeley, "Major Depressive Disorder in Older Adolescents: Prevalence, Risk Factors and Clinical Implications," *Clinical Psychological Review* 18, no. 7 (1998): 765–94.

cents; older youngsters tend to suffer from delusions more frequently than hallucinations. Delusions or hallucinations in adolescent depression seem to be uncommon, but, when they are present, they seem to signal an especially severe illness.

MORE ON ADOLESCENCE

The first person to formulate a psychological theory of adolescence was the American psychologist and educator G. Stanley Hall, who believed that emotional turmoil and crisis were always characteristic of this developmental period, something to be endured rather than understood. Writing at the beginning of the twentieth century, Hall proposed that the entire history of the human race had become part of each individual's genetic endowment and that the psychological development of each individual retold the story of human history. Borrowing a German phrase used to describe the sweeping romantic sagas of Schiller and Goethe, Hall characterized adolescence as a period of *Sturm und Drang*, "storm and stress," a phrase that was used to characterize adolescence for decades afterwards. Hall saw adolescence as a recapitulation of the conflicts of preindustrial civilization: a time of crusades and revolutions, great chivalry and great cruelties, self-sacrifice and brutal domination, fervent loyalty and unscrupulous treachery. Adolescents passed through a time of rapidly changing moods and emotions, unbridled optimism giving way to despair, melancholy alternating with youthful exuberance, before a mature, rational adult emerged from the chaos. Even after the "genetic" and historical components of Hall's ideas had been discredited, his concept of inevitable emotional storminess during adolescence persisted, becoming incorporated into psychological theories that followed and even into popular thinking about adolescence.

It turns out that the "storms" most adolescents go through are fairly minor and short-lived — perhaps better thought of as passing cloudbursts. Surveys of teens and their parents through the 1960s and 1970s indicated that adolescents generally tend to have positive self-concepts and place high value on the approval of their parents and that, while some bickering between teens and their parents about such everyday issues as what clothing they wear and what time to be in at night is common, serious conflict is not the norm. Sir Michael Rutter, a British child psychiatrist who has extensively researched and written about adolescent issues for several decades, puts it this way: "It is evident that normal adolescence is *not* characterized by storm, stress and disturbance. Most young people go through their teenage years without significant emotional or behavioral problems. It is true . . . that there are challenges to be met, adaptations to be made, and stresses to be coped with. However, these do not all arise at the same time and most adolescents deal with these issues without undue disturbance."[2]

A theory of adolescence that has better withstood the test of time is that of the great American psychologist Erik Erikson, who invented the term *identity crisis* in the 1960s to characterize the uncertainty, self-questioning, and existential confusion he believed was inevitable during adolescents' search for their place in the world.

Erikson's concept of the "identity crisis" of adolescence still remains one of the best formulations of these issues. Although the word *crisis* conjures up a meaning of danger and even possible catastrophe, Erikson's use of the word is more like that of the Chinese, encompassing a meaning of "opportunity" as well. "Turning point" might capture the idea better. According to Erikson, the main issue that confronts and preoccupies adolescents is a search for their identity as a person.

Erikson's theory has roots in psychoanalysis but emphasizes the interplay between the individual and society. You may be familiar with the "Eight Stages of Man," which he devised as the outline of his theory (see table 2-2). Each of Erikson's stages represents a developmental task that confronts the individual at a particular age as he or she confronts ever widening and complex social situations, expectations, and responsibilities. Erikson proposed

Table 2-2 The Life Cycle Stages Proposed by Erik Erikson

Stage	Age	Psychosocial Crisis
I	Infancy	Trust versus mistrust
II	Toddler	Autonomy versus shame and doubt
III	Preschool	Initiative versus guilt
IV	School age	Industry versus inferiority
V	Adolescence	Ego-identity versus role-confusion
VI	Young adulthood	Intimacy versus isolation
VII	Middle age	Generativity versus self-absorption
VIII	Old age	Integrity versus despair

that each stage has the possibility of a positive or negative outcome. If the individual is able to manage a positive outcome at any particular step, he or she moves on to the next with enhanced psychological coping and developmental tools. If the crisis is not well managed, the negative attribute will interfere with the next step in development and psychological problems are more likely.

Erikson postulated that adolescence is the first time a person begins to ask herself, in a serious way, "Who am I?" Also pressing for attention are the related questions, "Where did I come from?" "What do I want to become?"

Bodily changes—physical growth, hormonal changes, the onset of menstruation in girls, and voice change in boys—force the adolescent to come to terms with a new body image. Experimentations with the use of cosmetics in girls, with facial hair and body building in boys, and with clothing and hairstyles their parents don't approve of in both sexes (not to mention piercings and tattoos) are adolescents' efforts to discover their bodies and attempts at self-invention and self-definition.

During this time, greater psychological development allows adolescents to interact in more sophisticated ways with others, and they become much more preoccupied with what others think about them, often comparing these perceptions with how they feel about themselves. This may explain why teens seem determined to be centers of attention but simultaneously complain of feeling as if they are constantly being scrutinized and are "on stage." They crave feedback but at the same time are worried about what they might hear about themselves. As adolescents seek roles and models outside the home, the peer group becomes increasingly important as a reference point and sounding board. Idolization of athletes, musicians, and movie stars is part of this search for self-definition and also part of developing a vocational identity and the beginnings of thinking about career.

Sexuality is another aspect of personal identity that adolescents begin to explore, and exploration of the physical aspects of sexuality is only part of the process. Crushes and infatuations with unobtainable partners occur, with inevitable disappointment. The teenager may establish a sense of identity through couple-hood: "Who am I? I'm her boyfriend." Relationships are often not about sexual exploration so much as the youth's exploration of his own unformed identity as projected through the eyes of a beloved—the personal feedback of the youthful love affair helps the adolescent reflect on, redefine, and revise his image of himself. As Erikson explained it, "That is why many a youth would rather converse, and settle matters of mutual identification, than embrace."[3]

The adolescent's move towards autonomy and away from parental authority and control also means giving up some measure of parental protection and nurturance, often before secure and comfortable emotional self-reliance is possible. A stage of substituting dependence on a peer group for dependence on parents is not unusual, explaining the intense devotion among friends, cliques, and teams so often seen at this age. Extreme peer group conformity in choice of clothing styles, behavioral norms, even the heroes and idols of the group, provides acceptance and solidarity. Selection of foods and entertainment and use of language and slang expressions are in strict conformity to the peer group. Disdain, intolerance, and even cruelty towards those who act differently are common. This is a time when adolescents can become vulnerable to pathological group allegiances as well: gangs, religious cults, militaristic organizations—all groups that exploit the adolescent's tendency to view the world in terms of black and white. Teens may alternate between more independent and more dependent styles, perhaps even showing both simultaneously in different settings.

The possible negative outcome of this stage, *identity diffusion*, results in an individual who is constantly bedeviled by self-doubt and either morbidly preoccupied with the opinions of others or defiantly indifferent to them. Some adolescents attempt to escape feelings of alienation and anxiety by using alcohol and drugs. In his most comprehensive consideration of adolescence, *Identity, Youth, and Crisis*, Erikson summed up the dilemma of identity confusion by quoting Biff, a character in Arthur Miller's play *Death of a Salesman:* "I just can't take hold, Mom, I can't take hold of some kind of life."[4]

Like any developmental theory, Erikson's proposals about adolescence should not be taken as a blueprint for every individual. It is most important to remember that psychological development during adolescence is a process, not an event; it proceeds in fits and starts over a period of years (and of course, our search for the answer to the question "who am I?" is never really over at any age). Later theorists expanded and elaborated Erikson's ideas, emphasizing that the process is usually disorganized and erratic and that adolescents inevitably go through at least some periods of partial identity diffusion with its accompanying feelings of alienation.

The concept of *developmental foreclosure* has been proposed by American psychologist James Marcia to describe the process whereby the adolescent identifies and commits to some aspect of self-definition by incorporating the goals and values of others without the personal searching and self-examination inherent in true identity exploration.[5] The youth espouses the political or religious views of parents or significant others, sometimes fervently, but without an open exploration and consideration of alternatives. If, for some reason, some aspect of this "foreclosed" identity no longer fits, a temporary crisis can ensue until the adolescent readjusts or perhaps even reinvents this aspect of her identity. An adolescent who has unquestioningly accepted the teachings of the church she was raised in may be forced to question her allegiance to the denomination if she finds her developing political or social ideology at odds with its dogma. A period of questioning, searching, and perhaps stress and confrontation ensues before one or the other jarring element of identity is adjusted.

Inevitably, all this testing, exploring, questioning, and adjusting is psychologically stressful. The adolescent suffers disappointments in relationships, disillusionment with cherished ideas or values, frustration that the answer to "who am I?" keeps changing, anxiety that the answer to "what do I want to become?" isn't as clear as it seemed during childhood. It should not be surprising, then, that anxiety and low mood are common in adolescence.

Michael Rutter and his colleagues studied thousands of children and adolescents on England's Isle of Wight in an attempt to measure the frequency of psychological symptoms and illnesses in the population. They found that more than two-fifths of the 14- to 15-year-old boys and girls they interviewed reported substantial feelings of misery or depression. As Rutter concluded, "It seems that feelings of misery and depression are particularly common during adolescence and are more frequent during this age period than during either earlier childhood or adult life."[6] Many other studies have come up with similar findings.

What can we make of all this "misery" in adolescents? We know from similar studies (discussed below) that only a fraction of these adolescents have severe depression or mood disorders. Rather than depression, it may be more accurate to say that adolescents are prone to periods of *demoralization*.

In his classic book about psychotherapy, *Persuasion and Healing*, Johns Hopkins psychiatrist Jerome Frank states, "A person becomes demoralized when he finds that he cannot meet the demands placed on him and cannot extricate himself from his environment." Demoralized persons are "conscious of having failed to meet their own expectations or those of others, or of being unable to change the situation or themselves."[7] Where could we read a better description of adolescents' dilemma? Repeatedly finding themselves in strange new situations loaded down with expectations from parents, peers, and themselves, and often feeling powerless to affect the outcome, adolescents face big questions.

"In order to function," Frank states, "everyone must impose an order and regularity on the welter of experiences impinging upon him. To do this, he develops out of his personal experiences a set of . . . assumptions about himself and the nature of the world in which he lives, enabling him to predict the behavior of others and the outcome of his own actions."[8] This set of assumptions is called one's *assumptive world*. When something happens that disrupts a person's assumptive world, the environment suddenly seems unpredictable and a little scary. The individual may react with anxiety, feelings of loss of control, feelings of being trapped, powerless, and, yes, miserable and depressed for a time—the state of affairs that Frank calls demoralization.

In the process of identity development, adolescents' assumptive world is constantly being upset and jostled by new experiences that can throw it into doubt. They spend weeks getting up the courage to ask out on a date someone they think is just right for them, only to be turned down ("Maybe I'm not as good-looking/popular as I thought"). They fail an exam ("I'm not as smart as I thought"), or don't make the team ("not as athletic . . ."), or lose the audition ("not as talented . . ."). Even positive accomplishments like getting good grades can raise questions about negative identities ("I must be a nerd"). Adolescents often assume that what happens to them indicates something about what kind of person they are. They react strongly to disappointments and setbacks, because they wonder what such events indicate about who they are and what their future will be like. A slight setback that adults would react to with only minor disappointment often causes adolescents to feel much more upset and disappointed and to question themselves in very profound ways.

Reading through this, you might wonder why more adolescents don't need treatment for symptoms of demoralization. But as Rutter puts it, these challenges, adaptations, and stresses "do not all arise at the same time"; that is, only under rare and unusual circumstances is the adolescent faced with so many crises simultaneously that they overwhelm psychological resources to cope.

Jerome Frank developed his concept of psychological demoralization in the course of doing research on the effectiveness of psychotherapy. He studied persons with demoralization symptoms such as depression and anxiety so severe that they sought professional psychological treatment. As Frank discovered, the crucial elements that make psychotherapy effective for these individuals are surprisingly simple: patients must have faith that the therapist cares about them and knows how to help them. Fortunately, most teens have any number of persons in their life who meet these requirements; they are surrounded by concerned, supportive, and experienced persons—parents, teachers, coaches, clergy, even older friends, the list could go on and on—who can help them through periods of uncertainty and discouragement about themselves.

All adolescents go through periods of discouragement, suffer from occasional feelings of not fitting in, and are bothered by uncertainty about the future. We must be careful not to "medicalize" this growth process (as Anna Freud is guilty of doing, exemplified by her comment that "to be normal during the adolescent period is by itself abnormal"),[9] and we must remember that a majority of the teenagers in the studies by Rutter and others did *not* report undue depression or "misery."

WHEN IS DEPRESSION "SERIOUS"?

At this point, you may be a little confused. I told you earlier that depression is a serious illness, but just spent several pages telling you that adolescent complaints of being "miserable" are not uncommon and do not represent *clinical* depressions—that is, they do not usually warrant medical treatment. The way to understand this better is to recall the discussion in chapter 1 about depression the *symptom* and depression the *syndrome*. In this chapter, I've put an even finer distinction on the issue and have talked about the difference between *depression* and *demoralization*. But how are these related? Can one cause the other? Blend into the other? Where does intense demoralization end and the depressive syndrome begin?

At this point in time, the answers to these questions are simply not known. We know it is not uncommon for adolescents to pass through periods of "miserableness" quite unscathed. But we know that some of this miserableness is a prelude to, or an aspect of, a mood disorder. We also know that adults with mood disorders can have an episode of serious depression triggered by psychological stress and demoralization.

The big mistake that people make in deciding whether to seek treatment for a person with depression is to think that if he seems to have "real" reasons to be depressed, he won't need treatment because he'll "get over it" as soon as he deals with those reasons. A related error is thinking that this individual needs counseling or therapy but not medical treatment. This is not too different from the middle-aged man with chest pains trying to persuade himself that "it's only heartburn" rather than going to the nearest emergency room. When an individual has the signs and symptoms of the syndrome of depression, it's time to get professional help, not to try figuring out whether he has "reasons" to be depressed.

Because we have several ways of understanding depression, one perspective based on biology and the disease model, and a second perspective based on psychology and understanding how people react to events in their lives, it's tempting to think we should be able to categorize depressions in the same way: "biological" and "psychological." I've already led you into this way of thinking a bit, with the discussion of *depression* differentiated from *demoralization*. If only an understanding of people were so easy!

This categorizing of depressions works fairly well in some clear-cut cases at the extremes of the categories. No one would say that a teenage football player who sulks and broods for a day or two after his team misses a chance to be in the state playoffs is suffering from a mood disorder. Not much "biological" going on there. No one would say that Charlie from chapter 1 is simply discouraged, suffering from "normal" teenage angst. This boy is clearly ill.

But there is a large area between these extremes, where differentiation between "biological" and "psychological" depressions is not only impossible but also probably meaningless. Another great student of human behavior, Alfred Kinsey, the pioneering researcher on sexuality, said, "The world is not divided into sheep and goats . . . Nature rarely deals with discrete categories. Only the human mind invents categories and tries to force facts into separated pigeonholes."[10] Our mental lives involve a complex interplay between biology and psychology that is very poorly understood and probably cannot be teased apart. One set of forces affects the other, and there are probably complex feedback loops and an intertwining of influences and processes that make attempts to do so futile.

Michael Rutter, in talking about "causes" of psychological problems, makes the point that this entanglement of causation is also apparent in physical illnesses as well: we know that a germ called the tubercle bacillus causes tuberculosis. But we also know that genetic factors play a role in resistance to infection and to some extent determine who gets infected. We know, too, that nutritional status is important, that malnourished individuals are much more vulnerable to TB, making it in some ways an illness of poverty. To say that poverty causes tuberculosis isn't quite correct, but to say that tuberculosis is caused by a germ and leave it at that omits a lot of factors that need to be identified in order to treat the illness. Talking too much about what is "biological" and what is "psychological" in depression is simply a waste of time. Serious depression is both.

Not too long ago, psychiatrists and psychologists made the mistake of relying too much on theories to guide their treatment of depressed patients and not enough on research data and experience. We spent too much time trying to understand depressed persons rather than diagnosing and treating mood disorders. We now know that serious depressive syndromes must be treated medically and that psychotherapy alone will usually not make the patient better. But we also know that people with depressive illnesses are usually demoralized and need support, encouragement, education, and guidance. Adolescents with serious depression should not be denied either kind of treatment just because the details of their symptoms seem to suggest that either depression or demoralization predominates.

So, back to the original question posed earlier: what constitutes *serious* depression? Although you really need a medical or psychology degree and years of clinical training to be able to answer this question for any given individual, you can get some sense of what serious depression is like by rereading chapter 1 for the details of the depressive syndrome. Also, there are some red flags that should always make parents worry that their teen might be seriously depressed:

— *Persistent change in mood*: gloominess, sadness, grouchiness, or irritability that persists over several weeks, on more days than not, such that the teenager seems consistently different from her usual self
— *Loss of interest and enjoyment* in most of the activities that the adolescent usually spends time doing
— *Persistent changes in sleep habits and appetite*: complaints of insomnia, sleeping too much, loss of appetite or increased appetite that results in a weight change of ten pounds or so, persistent complaints of tiredness or low energy, looking tired or haggard all the time
— *Change in self-attitude*, that is, a change in the way the adolescent feels about himself: feeling worthless or useless, self-critical statements about not being as good as other kids, feeling that he is lazy, stupid, ugly, a failure, or good-for-nothing
— *Falling grades*, loss of concentration, complaints that schoolwork is suddenly more difficult
—*Preoccupation with death or illness, thoughts of suicide*

The next step in understanding adolescent depression is to learn about the different disorders that exhibit the depressive syndrome. Several decades of research have led to our current classification of the various mood disorders. The depressive syndrome shows up in all of them, but the severity and pattern of the depressive symptoms, their course over time, and some associated symptoms indicate that they are probably different illnesses. Research has also shown that the treatments of these different disorders sometimes need to be very different.

In the next chapter, I discuss the mood disorders of adolescence.

CHAPTER 3

The Mood Disorders of Adolescence

When psychiatrists and psychologists started thinking about serious depression as an illness and began to do research on the symptoms of depression, the course of the illness, and its response to various treatments, they found that serious depression shows up in different forms. These forms differ in severity and types of symptoms and in the timing of symptom development. This research has resulted in our current classification system of mood disorders.

PSYCHIATRIC DIAGNOSIS

Diagnosis is just as important in treating emotional problems as it is in treating physical illnesses. Diagnostic classification has two purposes in medicine: (1) to make predictions about the course of an illness and (2) to aid the clinician in selecting the treatment most likely to be effective. In the practice of psychiatry, since the physical basis for most psychiatric illnesses has yet to be discovered, classification systems are largely derived from studying groups of patients with different combinations of symptoms and seeing whether the different groups vary in the course of their illness or in their response to medications.

As different types of medications have become available to treat mood disorders, the classification system of mood disorders has continued to evolve. In this chapter, I describe various subtypes of mood disorders. These are the subtypes that currently seem to make sense to clinicians, because they serve one of the two purposes of diagnosis mentioned above: (1) they allow for a better prediction of the course of the illness, and (2) they allow for a rapid selection of effective therapy—saving the patient time that would be wasted on a trial of an ineffective medication.

At least once a month, it seems, I see a patient who requests to be "tested for clinical depression," the implication being that a blood test of some type will be able to detect the "chemical imbalance" that underlies serious mood problems. It's not an unreasonable request. Unfortunately, it's not a request that can be satisfied—not just yet. We don't have a blood test or x-ray or biopsy that can make the diagnosis of a mood disorder (or, for that matter, that can be used to confirm the diagnosis of most problems that psychiatrists treat).

This is because the biological and chemical basis of mood disorders remains a nearly complete mystery—no one knows what to test for. Despite literally hundreds of years of examining the bodily fluids and brain tissues of individuals with mood disorders, first with the naked eye, then with microscopes, then with x-rays and scanning devices, and more recently with incredibly sophisticated biochemical probes, no one has been able to find any abnormalities that can be accurately and reliably measured in people with this illness and used to aid in the diagnosis of these disorders. Although work on the genetics of mood disorders holds the promise that genetic markers for the illness may be discovered in the not too distant future—suggesting that a blood test might be possible that will identify at least some cases of the illness—and although some individuals with mood disorders have been identified as having subtle brain-scan abnormalities—again suggesting a possible diagnostic tool—the clinical applications of these findings are still far off. Modern psychiatrists are left with the same diagnostic tools available to nineteenth-century psychiatrists: their eyes and ears.

We psychiatrists listen to patients and their family members describe symptoms. What has changed? What doesn't feel right? When did it start? Do the symptoms come and go or stay all the time? We observe the patient for the signs of mood disorders described in chapter 1 by performing a *mental status examination,* the psychiatrist's equivalent of the physical examination. This consists of observing speech patterns and behavior, questioning about mood and thinking processes, and evaluating other aspects of mental functioning such as concentration and memory. After this process of history taking and examination, a picture of the person, of her symptoms and the course of her troubles, emerges. We identify a particular diagnostic category that seems a good fit with the clinical information, and once this is done, we can make predictions about the future course of the symptoms and, perhaps more importantly, select a treatment that has a good chance of relieving them.

MAJOR DEPRESSIVE DISORDER

Major depressive disorder is the name given to the mood disorder characterized by the development of the full-blown depressive syndrome. Research indicates that major depressive disorder is the most common mood disorder of adolescents and young adults.[1]

The illness usually has a fairly definite beginning, and, over a period of weeks, the various symptoms of depression gradually come over the adolescent one by one until the full syndrome is present. The symptoms can last for months, with studies indicating that seven to nine months is typical.[2] The symptoms can vary tremendously in severity from fairly mild symptoms that affect the teen's level of functioning only mildly to severe cases in which social, school, and home life are all severely affected.

In chapter 1 we met the parents of Charlie, who was showing the typical symptoms and course of illness of major depression. Charlie's symptoms were low mood, withdrawal, low energy, sleep and appetite problems, loss of interest in his usual pursuits, feeling bad about himself—symptoms that came on gradually over a period of weeks and basically drained the spark out of this previously energetic, confident boy.

Sometimes, however, major depression can look rather different, especially when the mood change is irritable rather than low. In these adolescents, the irritable, miserable mood (psychiatrists often use the term *dysphoria*) is so disruptive to the adolescent's social world, especially the family, that other symptoms of major depression are obscured. Another case study will illustrate this.

▼
_____

Heather's mother tried not to worry when her bright and usually bubbly 15-year-old daughter seemed to spend more Saturday afternoons listening to music in her room and fewer with her friends at the mall. But when Heather dropped out of the choral society, Maggie knew something was wrong.

"It's no fun anymore," was Heather's explanation for dropping out of the student choir only a month before the spring concert. "It's really boring; that stuff

Table 3-1 Symptoms of Major Depression

Mood Symptoms
  Depressed mood
  Dysphoric mood
  Irritability
  Loss of ability to feel pleasure (anhedonia)
  Loss of interest in usual activities
  Social withdrawal
  Feelings of guilt or worthlessness
Cognitive (Thinking) Symptoms
  Poor concentration
  Poor memory
  Indecision
  Slowed thinking
  Thoughts of death, suicidal thinking
Bodily Symptoms
  Sleep disturbance
    Insomnia
    Hypersomnia
  Appetite disturbance
    Weight loss
    Weight gain
  Fatigue
  Headaches
Symptoms of Psychosis
  Delusional thinking
  Hallucinations

is for nerds anyway," she said with a shrug of her shoulders, when her mom asked about it.

This explanation didn't quite sit right with Maggie, but she could guess what the real reason might be. Heather had auditioned to be a soloist in the concert and had been very disappointed that she wasn't chosen to sing any of the solo pieces. The choir director had told her that she wasn't quite ready for solo work yet but urged her to audition again for the fall concert. The director had also started telling the girls who were having trouble with their parts to stand next to Heather on the risers. "Heather has a strong voice and great intonation; she'll help carry you until you get the part down better," she would tell them in front of Heather and the whole group.

Heather had at first seemed to get over her disappointment, but as the weeks went by it seemed singing was a chore rather than a source of joy and pride. "She didn't mean what she said about my having a good voice," Heather said angrily when Maggie reminded her of her music teacher's encouraging words when Heather announced that she'd quit the choir. "She said that to humiliate me in front of *everyone*." So saying, Heather burst into tears and ran up to her room.

"Heather's just going through a stage," Maggie's sister reassured her one afternoon when they met at the grocery store. "Don't you remember when my Matt dropped off the swimming team with hardly an explanation and started writing poetry at all hours of the night? Kids' interests change all over the place at this age. They're finding themselves, that's all."

"I don't know," Maggie replied warily. "Heather's interests haven't changed. She seems to have lost interest in *everything*. She got lower grades in two subjects on her last report card, and besides she's so . . . oh, I don't know, so *mean* all of a sudden."

"Mean?" her sister asked.

"Well, she's so sarcastic about everything. She has Beth in tears several times a week."

"Big sisters criticize little sisters all the time at this age. It makes them feel grown up."

"I don't know, Fran. Heather and Beth always got along so well. They've never been mean to each other."

"Heather's never been a teenager, either, Maggie," Fran soothed, patting Maggie's hand on the grocery cart. "And believe me, it gets worse when they're juniors; but you'll get through it somehow. Everyone does!"

Things did get worse. And much worse than Fran had predicted. There were screaming matches between Heather and her mother and father, Phillip, several times a week. Heather's grades continued to drop, and she took to spending most of her time in her room listening to music. Several times, Maggie had awakened in the middle of the night still hearing the music playing softly in Heather's room. She'd gone in to turn it off only to find her daughter still awake, sometimes in tears, but unable to say why she was crying.

Heather started coming in later than her curfew on weekends and often had alcohol on her breath.

Maggie and Phillip got a phone call from one of Heather's teachers warning that summer school might be a good idea if Heather wasn't able to turn her grades around. "I'm worried about Heather, and I think you should be too. Some of the answers on her tests make me think she's not concentrating in class like she should. She doesn't seem to be able to grasp the concepts this semester." But Heather flew into a rage when Maggie and Phillip told her about the call from her teacher. "And I will *not* go to summer school! Don't even think about it! I'll kill myself first!" she hissed ominously through clenched teeth.

Maggie felt alone and bewildered in dealing with her changed daughter. Her sister Fran shook her head sympathetically and suggested Maggie and Phillip go to "Tough Love" meetings. Phillip started staying later at the office to avoid the tension at home, and one night had only half-jokingly threatened to leave home "until she's 21 and a normal person again—I'll send you a check every month but you can call me when this part is *over*." Even 12-year-old Beth seemed to be out of the house most nights, needing to "study" with classmates. "I work better with someone else there," she explained sheepishly. "And it's hard to concentrate at home."

And there was no talking to Heather about much of anything. Maggie had made up her mind several times to make an appointment for Heather to see a therapist, but then things would go better for a day or two and she'd hope that the worst was over. And when things seemed to be getting worse, Maggie would become terrified at how Heather might react to the idea of seeing a mental health professional, and she would put the idea off "until she's in a better mood."

Late one evening, the phone rang. Maggie picked up the receiver expecting to hear Heather with her latest excuse for being out later than she should be. Instead, Maggie heard a woman's voice, a woman who seemed to be calling from some crowded place with phones ringing and some kind of beeping sound in the background.

"Mrs. McAllister? This is Ruth calling from the emergency department at St. Luke's Hospital." Maggie felt something in the middle of her chest drop to the soles of her feet. "We have Heather here and—"

"Oh my God, is she alright?"

"Yes, Mrs. McAllister, she's not hurt. There was a car accident, but Heather was not injured. She's fine physically, but—"

"Oh, thank God. We'll come right over to bring her home. Should we—"

"Well, ah . . . yes, you need to come over, but the doctor wants to talk to you about admitting Heather to the hospital."

"I don't understand. I thought you said she wasn't injured."

"No, she wasn't, but the psychiatrist thinks that she needs—"

"Psychiatrist? But what—"

"Heather drove off in her friend's car and ran off the road out by St. Mary's cemetery. The police found her passed out in the driver's seat with alcohol on her breath."

"Oh, God," was all Maggie could say.

"She was pretty alert by the time she got here, but the psychiatrist thinks she's very depressed. She wants to admit Heather at least overnight and see her in the morning, to see if she's still feeling suicidal."

"Depressed? Suicidal? But she's never—"

"Heather had two bottles of over-the-counter pills in her pocket and we think she was planning to take an overdose. These particular pills probably wouldn't have caused anything serious, but anytime someone tries to hurt themselves we need to—"

Maggie wasn't listening anymore. Depressed? But depressed people are sad and gloomy, Maggie thought, not like this. Why did they think Heather was depressed? She didn't have anything to be depressed about. Could not getting the solo part in the spring concert have caused all this? No, that made no sense at all.

"We'll come right away," she said, and hung up the phone.

Because Heather's problems seem at first glance so different from Charlie's, it doesn't seem possible that they have the same illness: major depression. But when we review Heather's symptoms, they're not really so different.

First, of course, there is the mood change. Heather is mostly irritable and dysphoric rather than suffering what we typically call a "low" mood. But the mood change is dramatic and pervasive, with her all the time, every day, week after week. Next, she's lost interest in school, in going with her friends to the mall, and she complains that singing is no fun any more; she's developed a loss of pleasure in things, which you might remember is called *anhedonia*. Heather is in her room alone much of the time and isn't sleeping at night. She's having crying spells frequently. Her teacher has noticed poor concentration, and her grades are dropping.

Heather feels bad about herself and doesn't think she's a good singer after all; she even thinks that the music teacher's compliments were some kind of sarcastic ploy meant to make fun of her. This misinterpretation of the reality of the situation is, in fact, the kind of idea that can become increasingly preoccupying and gradually turn into a *delusion*, a psychotic symptom in which a person has a preoccupying false belief.*

Noting Heather's use of alcohol is also very important in diagnosing her depression. Although substance use and abuse can certainly be "stand alone" problems in adolescents or in adults, sometimes substance abuse problems get started and are sustained by a mood disorder and can be understood as secondary to it. The start of alcohol misuse (and anything that approaches regular use is *misuse* in adolescents) accompanied by the other symptoms are a strong indicator of the seriousness of Heather's problems. And, lastly, the serious attempt to harm herself carries a lot of weight and puts her collection of symptoms squarely into the category of major depression.

Because of her mostly irritable rather than depressed mood state, and because of her outwardly directed disruptive behaviors, especially towards her family, a superficial appraisal of Heather's situation might suggest that her problem is being *bad* rather than *sad*. But remember that the diagnosis of the syndrome of depression requires looking at many aspects of emotional life and behavior in addition to mood, and when this kind of survey is done with Heather, we come up with quite a list: a pervasive mood change, withdrawal from friends and family, low energy, poor concentration, sleep problems, loss of interest in usual pursuits, feeling bad about herself (to the point that she thinks life just isn't worth it and she tries to harm herself)—virtually the same list as Charlie's. Heather's diagnosis is the same as well: major depression.

No one is quite sure why this irritable mood is more common in adolescents than in adults. Irritability can certainly be a part of the picture in adults, but it is rarely the most prominent aspect of the mood syndrome as it can be in adolescents. Research shows that irritability as an expression of severe depression is most striking during adolescence. The symptoms

---

*Remember that, in mood disorders, the content of delusional beliefs is depressing in some way. In *A Mind That Found Itself*, written in the nineteenth century, author Clifford Beers describes his battle with a mental illness that was almost certainly a mood disorder. In one scene, he describes how, on a train ride to the psychiatric hospital, he noticed people standing on the station platforms reading the newspaper as the train passed through. Beers relates how convinced he was at the time that they were reading about *him*, about his long history of mental illness and about what a failure he had been. These themes of shame and failure are typical of a mood disorder.

of severe depression in children (under the age of 12) more closely resemble depression in adults, with low mood and energy level. Thus, the mood change that takes place in severe depression before and after adolescence can be different from that seen during adolescence. Why?

It is tempting to speculate that the struggle for independence and separation from family that preoccupies most adolescents somehow makes them more "prickly" and reactive in their interactions with parents and authority figures. Perhaps depression exaggerates the tendency towards defiance that is part of every teenager's drive to find and assert his independence. This theory would state, then, that psychological issues particular to adolescence shape the depressive feelings and result in the prominent irritability. But this is pure speculation, and this very important question remains unanswered.

Onset of a depression following a loss or disappointment of some type is not uncommon. In Heather's case, the disappointment was a rather minor one, and this is actually *not* typical. More commonly the loss is a significant one, such as the death of someone close, parental divorce, or the breakup of a serious relationship. The exposure to the suicide of someone close has been strongly linked to the development of major depression in adults. One might want to conclude from these sorts of data that loss and stressful events can cause major depression, but this conclusion would not be quite correct, for several reasons. First, some adolescents who get depressed do not seem to have a significant stressful event preceding the development of their depression. Second, many teens who suffer a significant loss do not go on to develop severe depression. A 1995 study compared the occurrences of stressful life events in teenagers with and without major depression. It found no statistically significant difference in the total number of stressful events in the two groups.[3] One expert on the relationship between depression and stressful events put it this way: "Undesirable events are . . . neither necessary nor sufficient to explain the onset of an episode of depression."[4] It's possible that rather than "causing" depression, stress and especially loss trigger the development of a depression in an adolescent who is vulnerable in some way, perhaps because of genetic factors (more on genetics in chapter 14).

How common is major depression in adolescents? We know from many studies on large groups of adolescents that between 15 and 20 percent of adolescents report that they've had symptoms that would warrant a diagnosis of major depression at some time in their life (this is known as the *life-*

time prevalence rate).[5] This is about the same rate that adults report, which has been interpreted to mean that adult major depressive disorder is an illness that starts in adolescence.

You may have noticed that I have used two similar-sounding terms: major depressive *episode* and major depressive *disorder.* Is there a difference? The answer to this question takes us into a discussion of the course that mood disorders take. We talk about "episodes" of mood disorders because they are illnesses that usually come and go throughout a person's lifetime. A person with major depressive disorder has an illness that takes the form of periods of time during which he has all the symptoms that make up the depressive syndrome: these periods are the major depressive episodes. Put another way, major depressive *disorder* is a psychiatric illness characterized by recurrent major depressive *episodes.*

Research has shown that in children and adolescents, a major depressive episode lasts, on average, approximately seven to nine months. [6] But a percentage of these youngsters have episodes that last longer; a small percentage will still have symptoms one to two years after the beginning of their illness.

Another very striking fact about adolescent depression is its tendency to recur. In one study of adolescents with major depression, over a period of three years researchers checked in with sixty-five patients who'd had an episode of major depression, meeting with each adolescent and his or her parents for an initial interview, then six months, one year, two years, and three years later. This study found that 54 percent of the adolescents experienced another episode of depression within the three-year period.[7] Other studies suggest that for adolescents who have had major depression, up to 70 percent will go through another period of major depression within the next five years.[8] The patients in these studies are usually from clinics and hospitals, so the results tend to show what the more severe forms of the illness can be like. Also, the studies often do not take treatment into account. The teens in some of these studies were getting only psychotherapy, some were taking medication as well, and some were getting little or no treatment. (That many teens with serious depression, even after getting a diagnosis by a professional, either never get into treatment or stop treatment after a short period of time is a finding in study after study of this type.)

These numbers are sobering. Major depressive disorder in adolescents can cause lengthy periods of symptoms, and once an adolescent has had an episode, the risk for recurrence is high.

DYSTHYMIC DISORDER

Like many words used in the field of medicine, *dysthymia* comes from Greek roots. The prefix *dys-* is from a word that means "bad" or "difficult," and the root *thymia* comes from the Greek word for "mind." In psychiatry, the meaning of this root word has altered a bit and usually refers to "mood." Dysthymia, then, is an illness characterized by "bad mood." How is it different from major depressive disorder?

Persons with dysthymic disorder suffer from a smoldering low-grade depressive syndrome that persists over a period of many months, sometimes for years. It is an illness that can remain undetected and thus untreated for a very long time. These individuals sometimes see a psychiatrist for the first time as adults, when they finally come to realize that the bad feelings they have constantly struggled against are *not* normal. When asked how long they have felt depressed, many of these patients say, "As long as I can remember." Because the symptoms can develop insidiously and smolder on without precipitating a crisis, dysthymic individuals can lose track of the onset of their depressed feelings and eventually seem to forget what "normal" feels like.

▼ ──────────────────────────────────────

Max was the most serious-looking 13-year-old I had seen in a long time. His khakis, white shirt, and blue-striped tie added to this impression, making him look almost like a little college professor rather than a young teenager.

"Max really didn't want to come today, doctor," his mother was saying. "But he said he would as long as he didn't have to miss school to come to the appointment."

"Why was that, Max?" I asked. "Kids don't often mind missing an hour or two of school, even if it is a trip to the doctor's office."

"I don't want to have to explain to people," he answered. "Other kids are too nosy about stuff. I didn't want to have to deal with a lot of questions."

Mrs. Phelps filled in Max's story. She had noticed her youngest son becoming more and more miserable over a period of many months. "He mopes around the house or sits and watches television. His grades have slipped again this year and—"

"No they haven't," Max said with a bit of irritation showing in his voice.

"Yes, they have, Max," his mom said. "You went from a 3 to a 2 in English in December." Mrs. Phelps looked up at me. "Now I know that's not a bad grade by any means. But it's the pattern we're worried about. He has dropped a grade point in at least one subject every semester for the past two years. Maybe it's not exactly a drastic drop, but his performance has been drifting downward for months." She looked over at her son. "Don't you agree, Max?"

"I guess so," he said looking down.

"Have you noticed any sleep problems or eating problems?" I asked.

"No, not particularly," Mrs. Phelps replied.

"Max?" I asked.

"Huh?" He said.

"Max, honey, talk to the doctor," his mom said soothingly. She looked up at me. "He doesn't seem to be paying attention half of the time. Do you think this might be why his grades are dropping?"

"I don't know why you have to say that over and over again," Max said. "It really makes me angry."

It turned out that anger was becoming more and more of a problem as well. Max was persistently defiant at home, often about little things. "Max made his bed every day almost from the time he started kindergarten. I don't think he's made it for a year. Now, I know a lot of boys his age don't, but it just doesn't seem right for Max. He's always been so eager to help around the house."

"How is Max getting along with his friends?" I asked.

"OK," Max responded.

I looked over at Max's mom. "Yes?" I asked.

"Well, it's hard for me to tell," she said. "He spends plenty of time with his friends, but he seems to worry a lot that nobody likes him."

"Mom!" Max said a little sharply.

"Max, honey, I'm just telling the doctor what you've told me so he can help you to feel better."

Max peered down at his shoes with a stony look.

"He just seems so miserable all the time," Max's mom said. "I see his friends run up the street yelling and laughing, and then Max comes along after them almost shuffling his feet, like it's almost too much effort. He wasn't this way before." Mrs. Phelps looked over at her son wistfully. "I remember him on his tenth birthday, so full of fun and energy. But something's changed; something has been creeping up on him for a long time now. It's happened so slowly that I didn't realize it for a long time."

The "something" was depression, and the pattern was dysthymic disorder. "You did just the right thing to bring Max in," I said. "I think we can make this 'thing' go away."

I like the word *smoldering* to describe dysthymic disorder. And just as a gust of wind can fan a smoldering fire into flame, stress can inflame the illness and cause symptoms of irritability to flare up. Because the symptoms aren't usually as dramatic as those of major depressive disorder, they may be easier to miss, but dysthymia can be just as dangerous.

Dysthymia seems to have an earlier age of onset than major depression, and studies have shown that children as young as 5 years old can be affected. These young people have a gloomy, pessimistic, down mood and are often preoccupied with feeling unloved and left out. They feel bad about themselves and worry that they don't measure up in various ways.

In a 1994 study that attempted to contrast and compare the symptoms of dysthymic disorder and major depressive disorder, the dysthymic children were younger, had fewer guilty feelings, had less sleep or appetite disturbance, and didn't suffer from the severe loss of pleasure that is characteristic of major depression. Their mood symptoms (depressed and irritable mood) and feelings of being unloved and without good friends were about the same (see table 3-2).

One of the most significant findings of this study is that early-onset dysthymic disorder seems to be an indicator for problems with other, often more severe mood symptoms later in life. As with an episode of major depression, a diagnosis of dysthymic disorder is a predictor of increased risk for more problems with depression later in life. In the 1994 study, a group of children was observed over a period of up to twelve years, and during that time 80 percent of the children with dysthymia had another episode of a mood disorder. More than two-thirds of the fifty-five children with early-onset dysthymic disorder went on to have an episode of the more severe collection of symptoms of major depression. Most of the time, these children's symptoms worsened into major depression with no completely well time in between, a phenomenon that has been called *double depression*. In double depression, the more severe symptoms of major depression become superimposed upon symptoms of dysthymia. In this group, the second and third years after the beginning of dysthymic symptoms were the period of highest risk.[9] More than one in ten dysthymic children in the study went on to develop symptoms of bipolar disorder (discussed below).

These findings have been interpreted to indicate that dysthymic disorder might be best thought of as a subtype or precursor of other mood disorders and may not really be a separate mood disorder after all. These findings also give new meaning to the idea that dysthymia is a "smoldering"

Table 3-2 Depressive Symptoms in Children with Dysthymic Disorder and
Major Depressive Disorder

| Symptom | Percentage of Children Reporting the Symptom | |
	Dysthymic Disorder	Major Depressive Disorder
Depressed or sad mood	91.7%	80.0%
Feeling unloved	55.6	48.9
Feeling friendless	41.7	40.0
Irritability	55.6	71.1
Anger	63.9	62.2
Anhedonia	5.6	71.1
Guilty feelings	13.9	31.1
Social withdrawal	8.3	53.3
Impaired concentration	41.7	67.4
Thoughts of wanting to die	16.7	42.2
Reduced sleep	22.2	62.2
Reduced appetite	5.6	46.7
Fatigue	22.2	64.4
Disobedience	58.3	43.2

Source: Maria Kovacs, Hagop Akiskal, Constantine Gatsonis, and Phoebe Parrone, "Childhood-Onset Dysthymic Disorder," *Archives of General Psychiatry* 51 (1994): 365–74.

type of depression, as in many of these young patients the symptoms flare up into full-blown major depression or bipolar disorder.

How common is dysthymic disorder? From studies of large groups of children and adolescents, researchers have estimated lifetime rates for dysthymia of between 0.1 and 8 percent in young people.[10]

BIPOLAR DISORDER

Some people with severe depressions have other types of abnormal mood states in addition to their depressions, periods that are in many ways the opposite of depression. During these episodes, they experience increased physical energy and psychological agitation. Instead of being slowed down and lethargic, they feel sped up and energized. Their thoughts can speed up so much that their speech can't "keep up"; they jump from topic to topic and they don't make sense. Their mood state can be giddy and high, or very irritable. But whether the abnormal mood state is pleasantly high or irrita-

Table 3-3 Symptoms of Mania

Mood Symptoms
   Elated, euphoric mood
   Irritable mood
   Grandiosity
Cognitive (Thinking) Symptoms
   Feelings of heightened concentration
   Accelerated thinking ("racing thoughts")
Bodily Symptoms
   Increased energy level
   Decreased need for sleep
   Erratic appetite
   Increased sexual feelings
Symptoms of Psychosis
   Grandiose delusions
   Hallucinations

ble, these individuals are abnormally energized, restless, and activated. These are some of the symptoms of *mania*.

People with bipolar disorder can also have a strange mix of the activation and agitation of mania combined with the negative thinking and mood of depression, a separate mood state called a *mixed affective state*, or simply a *mixed state*. Mixed states are very dangerous, because depressing thought patterns are combined with excess energy, restlessness, and an inner sense of pressure and tension. This negative energy puts these individuals at high risk for hurting themselves with suicidal behaviors.

Originally, the name for the illness characterized by periods of depression and periods of manic symptoms was *manic-depression* (or *manic-depressive illness* or *disorder*). More recently, the term *bipolar disorder* has come into fashion, taking its name from the fact that, in this illness, people suffer from abnormal mood states that are the polar opposites of each other: depression and mania.

Bipolar symptoms can be dramatic and extremely dangerous. But they can be rather subtle as well. Individuals may not have the frenzied, disorganizing extreme mood state of mania but may instead have *hypomania* ("mania," with the Greek prefix meaning "below"), a less severe "high" in which they are overconfident, tend to be reckless and lose inhibitions, and have a giddy overoptimism that causes them to take unaccustomed risks and exercise poor judgment. Some people cycle through different moods almost on a daily basis, being gloomy then giddy then irritable for brief periods of time with hardly any periods of normal mood. These variations on the bipolar theme are well described in adults, but not in adolescents. Psychiatry is only beginning to understand how these illnesses shown up in younger people.

For this reason, I've not attempted to sketch out a "typical" case history for bipolar disorder in young people. The course of the illness is tremendously variable and the symptoms vary greatly as well. The diagnosis should be considered whenever a young person's depressive symptoms include a great deal of irritability and hyperactivity or when there are dramatic shifts of mood from depressed to periods of overconfidence, uncharacteristic risk-taking behaviors, or elation. Symptoms might include intense temper tantrums that seem to come out of nowhere and go on for hours, spending sprees, uncharacteristic clowning, or giddiness that disrupts schoolwork.

The diagnosis and treatment of bipolar disorder in children and adolescents are further complicated by the similarity of manic and hypomanic symptoms to the symptoms of other psychological problems of adolescence. Adolescents with mild manic symptoms can have poor concentration, restless overactivity, and an inability to attend to and complete tasks that can resemble attention-deficit/hyperactivity disorder (ADHD; discussed in chapter 10). The irritability and temper tantrums of a depressed teenager can be difficult to separate from similar symptoms seen in mild bipolar disorders. These diagnostic problems lead to problems in choosing treatments. The stimulant medications used to treat ADHD (such as methylphenidate, brand name Ritalin) will make the symptoms of bipolar disorder worse. Antidepressant medications can also cause problems for persons with bipolar disorder, seeming to "push" depressed bipolar patients into hypomanic, manic, or mixed states. Psychiatrists currently are in agreement that there are three major subtypes of bipolar disorder: *bipolar I*, *bipolar II*, and *cyclothymia*.

Bipolar I

Bipolar I is the designation for the classic variety of bipolar disorder characterized by full-blown manic attacks and deep, paralyzing depressions. A schematic representation of the moods of bipolar I is shown in figure 3-1.

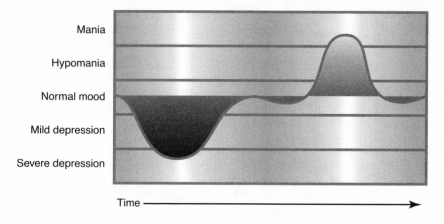

Mania

Hypomania

Normal mood

Mild depression

Severe depression

Time ⟶

Figure 3-1 Mood changes in bipolar I

The pattern of abnormal mood episodes seems to vary widely, and the pattern of the illness is almost as individual as the person who has the illness. Symptoms of bipolar I usually begin in the late teens or early twenties, so it is important to consider the diagnosis in young people with any type of mood disorder. Like the other mood disorders, bipolar I is what physicians refer to as a *relapsing and remitting illness*—during the course of the illness, its symptoms come and go of their own accord and may disappear, without any treatment at all, for months or even years at a time. Clinical studies on the course of bipolar disorder performed in the years before effective treatments for this disorder were available document and illustrate the pattern of bipolar disorder symptoms that existed when the illness was not treated—what physicians call the *natural history* of the illness.

In a 1942 study, researchers looked at the records of sixty-six patients with "manic-depressive psychosis," some of whom had been under observation for up to twenty-six years. These patients went through what we now call "episodes" of the illness, periods of severe depression or mania that lasted for several months (though sometimes much longer) and then went away on their own, with the patient's emotional state returning to normal. Although a few patients seemed to have had only one episode of illness in the period of the study, about a third had two to three episodes; a third, four to six episodes; and a third, more than seven. A few had twenty or more episodes (see table 3-4). Unfortunately, when a person is diagnosed with bipolar I disorder, there is no way to know whether the individual will have another two or three episodes during his or her lifetime or more than twenty.

Table 3-4 Episodes of Illness in Sixty-six Adult
Patients with Bipolar Disorder

Number of Episodes	Percentage of Patients
1	8%
2–3	29
4–6	26
More than 7	37

Source: Data from Thomas A. C. Rennie, "Prognosis in Manic-
Depressive Psychosis," *American Journal of Psychiatry* 98
(1942): 801–14; quoted in Frederick Goodwin and Kay Redfield Jamison, *Manic-Depressive Illness* (New York: Oxford
University Press, 1990), 133.
Note: This study was done before the availability of any effective treatment for bipolar disorder.

Bipolar I is the classic manic-depressive illness, with fully developed
manic episodes and episodes of severe depression, and is also characterized
by long periods of "hibernation," when the symptoms temporarily disappear. The number of episodes varies enormously, but individuals who have
only one or two episodes seem to be the exception rather than the rule. Before the availability of effective treatments, the average length of each
episode, if untreated, was about six months (in the 1942 study discussed
above, the average duration was about six and a half months), but episodes
that lasted years and years were not at all uncommon.

Bipolar I disorder seems to be uncommon in teenagers. In 1995, an important study on mood disorders in high school students was published in
the *Journal of the American Academy of Child and Adolescent Psychiatry.*[11]
To find out how common the various subtypes of mood disorders were in
high school students, these researchers interviewed 1,709 boys and girls between the ages of 14 and 17 who attended a high school in western Oregon.
The students were interviewed twice, about a year apart. Only two cases
of bipolar I were identified, that is, two students had a history of a full-blown
mania, the main diagnostic criterion for bipolar I.

Bipolar II

Bipolar II is characterized by fully developed depressive episodes and

Table 3-5 Features of Bipolar I Disorder

Mood
  Fully developed manic episodes
  Fully developed depressive episodes
Other Features
  Untreated episodes average six months

episodes of *hypo*mania. Figure 3-2 shows a schematic representation of the moods of bipolar II.

When lithium became available in the United States in the 1970s and researchers were trying to find better diagnostic criteria for bipolar disorder, several noticed a large group of patients who didn't have a history of fully developed manic episodes but who seemed to have a bipolar disorder nonetheless. These people had severe depressions, but their "highs" never developed into mania. Were they "manic-depressives" who were still early in the course of their illness and simply hadn't had time to have a fully developed manic episode? Several studies attempting to answer this question concluded that these patients did *not* usually go on to have fully developed mania. In one study, less than 5 percent of the patients with recurrent depressions and hypomania eventually became manic.[12] Several studies also showed that many patients with this type of disorder had relatives with a bipolar mood disorder also characterized by major depressions and hypomanias.[13] Although people with bipolar II sometimes have family members who have bipolar I or depressive disorders (without either mania or hypomania), the disorder frequently seems to show up in an identical form in affected families: family members of a person with bipolar II who have mood disorders also tend to have the bipolar II symptom pattern.[14] People with bipolar II disorder also seem to be at higher risk for alcoholism.[15]

Compared with people who have bipolar I disorder, those with bipolar II seem to have more problems with depression—in fact, the depression is sometimes so prominent that many receive a diagnosis of depressive disorder and don't get treatment for bipolar disorder at all. In a study from the National Institutes of Health published in 1995, 559 adult patients diagnosed with a *depressive* disorder were observed over time, some for up to eleven years. Almost 9 percent of them developed symptoms of bipolar II.[16] The first hypomanic episode usually could be documented within several months of the onset of severe depression, but sometimes it took up to nine

Figure 3-2 Mood changes in bipolar II

years for the correct diagnosis to become clear. Some of these 559 "depression" patients also developed a manic episode, that is, they actually had bipolar I, but this was far less common (only 3.9 percent). This study also found that patients with bipolar II disorder had longer depressive episodes (about a year) than those with bipolar I (about six months).

The study of Oregon high school students described above found eleven adolescents (about 0.6 percent) who had had a major depressive episode and had also gone through a period of elevated or irritable mood and other symptoms of hypomania, the pattern of bipolar II.[17] As you might already have figured out, this is about five times the number of students with bipolar I disorder. This finding is consistent with several studies in adults indicating that bipolar II may be more common than bipolar I.

Cyclothymic Disorder

Cyclothymic disorder, or cyclothymia, is characterized by frequent short periods (days to weeks) of depressive symptoms and hypomania separated by periods (which also tend to be short—on the order of days to weeks) of fairly normal mood. By definition, the person does not have either fully developed major depressive episodes or manic episodes. A schematic representation of the moods of cyclothymia is presented in figure 3-3.

Individuals with cyclothymic disorder have very frequent ups and downs of mood with only comparatively few periods of "normal" mood. Cyclothymic disorder also begins early in life—in the late teens or early twen-

Table 3-6 Features of Bipolar II Disorder

Mood
    Fully developed depressive episodes
    Hypomanic episodes
Other Features
    Increased sleep and appetite during depressions
    Depression sometimes more chronic
    Family history of bipolar II
    Later age at first hospitalization
    Fewer hospitalizations
    Possible increased risk for alcoholism

ties. Although many persons with this disorder never develop more severe mood symptoms, a significant number of them eventually have a fully developed depression or manic episode, that is, they develop bipolar disorder. In one study, about 6 percent of patients with the cyclothymic pattern eventually had a manic episode, putting them into the bipolar I category, but a higher number (25 percent) developed severe depression, that is, they turned out to have bipolar II.[18] However, perhaps half of people with the cyclothymic pattern never develop symptoms of "full-blown" bipolar disorder—a finding that makes cyclothymia a true diagnosis in its own right.

Family history studies suggest some relationship between cyclothymia and other bipolar disorders. People with cyclothymia often have relatives with bipolar disorder but rarely have relatives suffering from depressions only. Treatment experiences seem to confirm this relationship—the mood swings of cyclothymic disorder often respond to many of the same treatment approaches as the bipolar disorders. Cyclothymia was at one time thought to be a personality type, not an illness. Research indicates that this is not true.

In the Oregon study, 5 of the 1,709 students surveyed were diagnosed with cyclothymic disorder. These students had suffered from ups and downs of mood with periods of significant depression but had never experienced the full syndrome of a major depressive episode.[19]

Bipolar "Spectrum" Disorders

If you look at the end of the section on bipolar disorders in the American Psychiatric Association's *Diagnostic and Statistical Manual*, you will see a

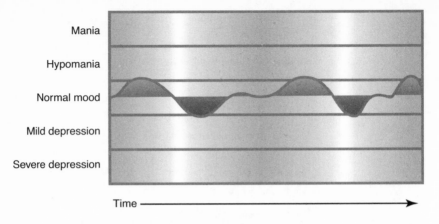

Figure 3-3 Mood changes in cyclothymia

category titled "Bipolar Disorder Not Otherwise Specified" (also called simply "bipolar NOS"). This odd category exists because the developers of the DSM recognized that there are patients who seem to have a kind of bipolar disorder but don't really fit the usual picture for bipolar I or II or cyclothymia.

Psychiatrists have long recognized the existence of many forms of bipolar disorder. For many years, clinicians have described various types of "soft" bipolar disorder, mostly in patients who came to be treated for depression and whose illness seemed related to bipolar disorder.[20] Terms such as *pseudo-unipolar depression* and *bipolar III* have been coined to describe various types of severe depressions that have some features of bipolar disorder but do not fall into traditional categories for bipolar diagnoses.

As more and more treatments for bipolar disorder become available and as more research on the mood disorders is done, we are finding that many patients who suffer from mostly depressive symptoms can benefit from treatment with medications for bipolar disorders and may, in fact, have a type of bipolar disorder. While we haven't yet figured out how to classify and accurately diagnose these problems, it is becoming clear that they are related in some way to bipolar disorders and that many depressed patients who don't seem to have classic "manic-depressive illness" benefit from medications used to treat those disorders.

Table 3-7 Features of Cyclothymic Disorder

Mood
   Frequent alteration between mild depression and mild hypomania
   Short irregular cycles (days)
   Only short periods of normal mood
Other Features
   Pattern appears in late teens, early twenties
   Frequently mistaken for problems with "personality"
   Sometimes develops into bipolar I or II disorder

MORE ON DIAGNOSIS

As you've probably noticed from the discussion thus far, the boundaries between the various depressive "disorders" of adolescence are not very clear. Studies indicate that children and adolescents with dysthymia can eventually develop major depressive episodes. Does it make sense to change such a child's diagnosis to major depressive disorder? Did one illness turn into another? Did the child have major depressive disorder all along? If so, why give the problem two different names?

Follow-up studies indicate that a large number of adolescents who have had a major depressive episode go on to develop symptoms of mania within a period of five years after the onset of their depressive symptoms. An informative study published in 2001 looked at seventy-two patients who had been treated for a major depressive episode as children (average age 10 years). When these individuals were contacted about ten years later (average age about 20 years), almost half reported having experienced manic or hypomanic symptoms.[21] As I mentioned above, about one in ten young persons who have had a diagnosis of dysthymia eventually develop bipolar symptoms. Should all patients with early-onset severe depressions be considered to have a bipolar disorder and treated accordingly?

The diagnostic classification of bipolar disorder in young people is a matter of great controversy. For many years, bipolar disorder was thought to be extremely rare in young people — even though research data on adults indicated that the first symptoms of bipolar disorder usually appeared before the age of 20. Perhaps because of a reluctance to diagnose children with an illness known to be a lifelong problem, and perhaps because of a hesitation to prescribe for children the powerful medications used to treat its symptoms, bipolar disorder in young children received little attention from researchers until quite recently.

More recent research is showing that bipolar disorder in children and adolescents may not be the same as bipolar disorder in adults, especially when the disorder has a childhood (rather than an adolescent) onset.

Research on bipolar disorder is beginning to show that it is probably not as rare in children as was once thought and that even very young children can have bipolar symptoms. In one study that looked at bipolar symptoms in the pediatric (under 18) age range, nearly a third of the patients were younger than 12 and the average age of onset for these young patients was 8½.[22] This same research is also shedding light on why psychiatrists used to think pediatric bipolar disorder was a rare diagnosis: bipolar disorder in children doesn't look the same as bipolar disorder in adults. If you look for adult symptom patterns in young children, you won't often see them.

When bipolar disorder occurs in young children (before puberty), it seems to be a more severe form of the illness. Perhaps this is because children who develop symptoms of bipolar disorder at so young an age seem to have a heavier genetic "loading" for mood disorders than do people with onset as adolescents or adults. Many children with bipolar disorder have more family members with mood disorders than do patients diagnosed as adults. For many of these children, both sides of the family have individuals with mood disorders. [23] Another difference between bipolar disorder in children and adults is that, rather than mania or hypomania, a major depression is frequently the first sign of the disorder in children. Several studies indicate that 20 to 30 percent of young people with major depressions go on to develop manic symptoms later in life.[24]

But the most striking difference between childhood-onset and later-onset bipolar disorder is the course of the illness. Pediatric bipolar disorder is a much more continuous illness than the adult form. In most adults, the illness usually appears in discrete episodes of depression or mania and the symptoms go into remission for months or years at a time. Children, on the other hand, often have long periods of continuous, rapid cycling: they sometimes cycle between depression and mania several times a day, having a laughing fit one moment and talking about wanting to shoot themselves the next.[25] One study of bipolar disorder in the pediatric age range described children who had more than a hundred "mini-manias" in a year, mood episodes that lasted only a day or two. In this study, none of the research subjects under the age of 9 had a single mood episode lasting two weeks or more as their only episode. In these children, a complex pattern of frequent, short episodes was the rule, not the exception.[26]

What do these findings mean for the adolescent age range? Will adolescents tend to show the clinical picture of the "adult" disorder or the childhood-onset disorder?

The answers to these questions are still not known, and the subspecialty of early-onset mood disorders is an area of psychiatry that is in tremendous flux. Behavioral scientists are still arguing over which diagnostic categories make sense and how the different categories are related to one another.

It is useful to remember that modern psychiatry's tendency to split different mood problems into separate diagnostic categories depending on symptom pattern and duration is comparatively new. In fact, the category of mood disorders as a subgroup of psychiatric disorders is only about two hundred years old. Before that, such words as *insanity* and *madness* were used very loosely to refer to almost any kind of severe psychiatric problems, even for illnesses we now recognize as medical illnesses that can cause psychiatric symptoms, such as central nervous system syphilis and Alzheimer's disease. The term *melancholia* was used to refer to illnesses we would call severe depression, but this was thought of as a type of "madness" too.

At the end of the nineteenth century, the great German psychiatrist Emil Kraepelin wrote a new edition of his influential textbook of psychiatry and coined the term *manic-depressive insanity* to encompass *all* the relapsing psychiatric disorders characterized by abnormal mood states. What we now call major depressive disorder, dysthymia, and the various types of bipolar disorder would have been considered forms of "manic-depression." Dr. Kraepelin believed that each of these illnesses was a variation of one illness: "In the course of years I have become more and more convinced that all [mood disorders] only represent manifestations of a *single morbid [disease] process*."[27] Kraepelin proposed that seemingly different mood disorders share the same fundamental causes and therefore can never be accurately separated into distinct categories. No one has yet proven Kraepelin's view incorrect; in fact, in European psychiatry, the broad category of "manic-depression" is still often used to encompass *all* mood disorders.

For parents wondering what treatment is best for their depressed child, this discussion might seem a rather useless debate about theoretical matters, the psychiatric equivalent of medieval theologians debating the number of angels that can dance on the head of a pin. But if you remember what I said previously about the importance of diagnosis in predicting the future course of an illness and helping select treatment, it becomes clearer that this "theoretical debate" has important practical implications. Research on treatments is meaningful only if the researchers agree upon the diagnosis of the individual being treated.

For a time after the first antidepressant medications became available, in the early 1960s, these medications were thought to treat just about any kind of depression. People who suffered from mild, moderate, or severe depressions, with or without the associated symptoms of the depressive syndrome, were often prescribed a "mood elevator," as these pharmaceuticals were sometimes called. The belief then was that antidepressants treated the symptom of depression no matter what the cause, just as aspirin will bring down a feverish person's temperature whether the fever is caused by the flu, pneumonia, or malaria.

Soon, it became apparent that antidepressants were of tremendous benefit to some people who complained of depression but seemed to have no effect on others, and also that the medications could cause some depressed individuals to develop a manic episode (those who, as we now realize, had a bipolar disorder). By studying the characteristics of patients for whom these medications did or did not work, it became possible to predict with better accuracy which patients antidepressants would help.

Now we have several dozen different antidepressants available, another half a dozen or so mood-stabilizing medications, plus several other classes of medications that seem to be helpful in some mood disorder patients. Unfortunately, we are still not very good at predicting precisely which medication will work best for which patient. One of the first steps in getting better at this is improving our diagnostic categories.

Another problem in trying to make a diagnosis in a young person is that mood disorders are, by their nature, relapsing and remitting disorders: symptoms develop, go on for a time, and then may go away on their own and without any treatment. As you have seen, our diagnostic categories are based on how the symptoms fluctuate over time. In a young person who is suffering from depressive symptoms for the first time, an accurate diagnosis may be impossible simply because the course of the illness hasn't had time to play out.

Despite these problems with diagnosis, there are a few facts most psychiatrists agree on. The division of mood disorders into two broad categories based on whether the individual has only depressive symptoms or has depressive as well as manic or mixed symptoms seems to be an important distinction. The terms *unipolar depression* and *bipolar depression* (or *disorder*) describe these two types of depression problems. The bipolar disorders have several subcategories as well, as I've described above. We have already seen that depressive disorders are further subdivided into *major depressive disorder* and *dysthymic disorder*. The foundation for medical treatment of unipolar depressions tends to be antidepressant medications, and that for bipolar disorders is usually a mood-stabilizing medication. But either type—or both types—of medication may be used in some patients with either type of disorder, because such combinations have been shown to be necessary and effective for some patients.

Some interpret this as proving that Dr. Kraepelin was right after all, that all the mood disorders stem from a "single morbid process." Others insist that we just haven't figured out the right system of categories and diagnostic methods.

So, what is the bottom line here? Psychiatric diagnosis is imprecise and difficult, and the making of a diagnosis must often be tentative. The diagnosis is helpful in predicting the probable course of the illness over time but less helpful in selecting a particular medication.

THE IMPORTANCE OF TREATMENT

Although mental health professionals may disagree about the classification of depressive disorders of adolescence, there is little disagreement about the importance of treatment. Three facts underscore the importance of getting treatment started quickly and making sure the youngster stays in treatment: (1) depression causes adolescents to suffer significant impairment in many areas of functioning; (2) serious depression is associated with other psychiatric problems, especially substance abuse; and (3) serious depression is a relapsing illness, and adolescent depression can lead to depression in adulthood.

One of the most important reasons for aggressive treatment of depressive disorders in adolescence is the tremendous toll these illnesses take on the functioning and development of teenagers if untreated. As you have seen in this chapter, the symptoms of these disorders can go on for many months, even years, if not treated.

The consequences are far more than repeating classes or being held back a year in school. These illnesses can essentially shut down the developmental process during a period of very important emotional growth and change. In chapter 2, I reviewed the developmental "tasks" of adolescence, essentially the struggle for differentiation from parents and establishment of a personal identity. Adolescence is a time when important groundwork is laid for mature social functioning and for educational and career development. The adolescent begins to learn to navigate independently in the world and to develop interpersonal skills such as negotiation and compromise. These require a strengthening of self-confidence and healthy independence, exactly the things the adolescent is deprived of by depression. A year of developmental "shutdown" can require several years of "catch-up" to overcome.

In a study that compared the school performance of sixty-two depressed adolescents (average age about 15 years) with thirty-eight adolescents who had no psychiatric illness, the depressed adolescents showed a variety of impairments.[28] In addition to lowered school achievement, these youngsters were more likely to have behavioral problems in school, they complained that they didn't like their teachers, and their parents received more teacher complaints about them—all illustrating how this illness poisons school life and relationships for the affected adolescent.

There is also evidence that a period of depression has long-lasting effects on adolescents even after they recover from an episode of the illness. The researchers who conducted the Oregon study discussed earlier found that depressed adolescents were "scarred" by the experience of depression in long-lasting ways.[29] They compared a group of students who had never been depressed with a group who had developed and recovered from a major depressive episode. When the adolescents were studied several months after the depressed students had recovered, problems with excess worrying and social withdrawal were found to be more common in the once depressed than in the never depressed group. The formerly depressed students also had less emotional independence and tended to need more emotional support and approval from others. And cigarette smoking was more common among the formerly depressed students. Perhaps the most instructive finding of this study was that only about a quarter of the adolescents who had gone through a depression had received treatment of any kind for their mood problems. One wonders whether, if more of these teens had gotten treatment and thus been depressed for a shorter period of time, depression's "scars" would have been milder and perhaps less frequently observed.

Another reason for aggressive treatment of depressive disorders in adolescents is the tendency for depressed adolescents to have other mental health problems, especially behavioral problems. In a study of sixty-seven adolescents with major depression, nearly one in six had behavioral problems severe enough to warrant the diagnostic label "conduct disorder."[30] Young people receiving this diagnosis have serious behavioral problems such as aggressiveness (bullying others and fighting), engaging in property destruction, stealing, truancy, and running away from home. Another study found that these types of severe conduct problems sometimes develop as a complication of the depression and persist even after the depressive symptoms go into remission.[31]

Perhaps the most serious problem associated with depressive disorders is substance abuse. The vignette about Heather illustrates just how dangerous a combination this is. Depressed adolescents, especially girls, are at higher risk than depressed adults for substance abuse, especially as they progress into early adulthood,[32] and the combination of problems puts adolescents at a much higher risk of suicidal behaviors than does either problem alone.

Lastly, the finding that adolescent depressive episodes predict problems with serious depression in adulthood further emphasizes the need for early identification and treatment. A 1995 study looked at the outcome of adolescent major depressive disorder in early adulthood by interviewing young adults who had participated in a study of adolescent major depression about seven years previously. The results were striking: more than two-thirds of the depressed adolescents had suffered at least one recurrence of major depression. Even more striking was the effect of recurrent depressions on the functional level of the young person. Individuals who had suffered multiple major depressive episodes in the previous years completed less schooling, reported less satisfaction with their lives and more impairment in relationships with friends, and scored lower on a functional rating scale. Also, more had become parents. The individuals who had not suffered a recurrence did not differ from a never depressed control group on any of these measures.[33] These findings show just how important it is to prevent recurrences of depression in adolescents.

CHAPTER 4

Mood Disorders

A Summary of Diagnostic Categories in the DSM

Parents who read a diagnosis in their child's medical records or insurance statements often have questions about the diagnostic categories used by mental health professionals and have concerns about the implications of various diagnostic terms. Psychiatry is one of the few medical specialties that have a more or less official list of disorders and diagnoses. In this chapter, we'll take a closer look at the latest version of this list, the fourth edition of the *Diagnostic and Statistical Manual of Mental Disorders* (the DSM IV), developed and published by the American Psychiatric Association. I present here a brief overview of the DSM and explain some of the diagnostic terminology for depressive and other mood disorders.

WHAT IS THE DSM?

The roots of the DSM IV go at least as far back as the United States Census of 1840, which included the category of "idiocy/insanity" in its classification system of American citizens. By 1880, there were seven categories into which persons with mental illness could be placed: mania, melancholia, monomania, paresis, dementia, dipsomania, and epilepsy.[1] In 1917, the American Medico-Psychological Association (the forerunner of the American Psychiatric Association) developed a statistical manual for use in mental hospitals that included various categories of diagnoses. As time went on, other organizations interested in the statistics of mental illness (such as the Veterans Administration and the United States Army) developed their own statistical manuals. The World Health Organization, after the Second World War, included a long section on mental disorders in the sixth edition of its *International Classification of Disease* (the ICD 6).

In 1952, the American Psychiatric Association published the *Diagnostic and Statistical Manual: Mental Disorders,* the DSM I. This work differed from previous statistical manuals because it contained a glossary that described the symptoms of the different disorders. Thus, in addition to containing an official list of categories of mental illness, the DSM I provided guidance to the clinician in making psychiatric diagnoses. By the time the third edition of the manual appeared in 1980 (the DSM III), each category of psychiatric disorders had a list of *diagnostic criteria*—a list of symptoms and other characteristics of each disorder that were thought to define it and to set it apart from other psychiatric disorders.

As its name now indicates, the DSM has become much more than a list of official diagnoses to be used to collect statistics on mental illness; it has developed into a valuable clinical tool that has proven immensely useful to clinicians and to those who do research on psychiatric illnesses. Now, when a patient goes to a new doctor and her medical records indicate a diagnosis of, say, "panic disorder" or "anorexia nervosa," the new doctor knows (if the last psychiatrist did his job well, of course) that the patient has had certain symptoms and not others and that the symptoms have troubled her for a certain period of time. Use of the DSM in research means that when you read in a study of some particular psychiatric disorder in a professional journal that "the patients met the DSM IV diagnostic criteria" for that disorder, you can be sure that all the patients in the study had a certain well-defined collection of symptoms and other characteristics in common and that the researchers are not mixing, as it were, psychiatric "apples and oranges."

Because the DSM contains a list of psychiatric diagnoses followed by succinct and clearly written criteria for making those diagnoses, it has the unfortunate effect of making psychiatric diagnosis look easy. It is tempting for individuals who do not have any psychiatric training to see the manual as a series of symptom checklists that can be easily applied to make the diagnosis of mental illness. This is not the case, for a number of reasons.

First of all, only with an enormous amount of training and experience can one gain an appreciation for the very wide range of *normal* emotions and behaviors and have a sense of what falls outside this normal range. Significant clinical experience and judgment are needed to decide what constitutes an *"irritable* mood" or an "increase in energy" that is *clinically* significant. The DSM is full of diagnostic criteria that use qualifiers—*"clinically significant," "marked* impairment," *"excessive* involvement in . . ."— all requiring judgment based on experience. Even some counseling and therapy professionals, if they have not trained in a setting where they have had the opportunity to see very sick patients, may not really have an appreciation for what constitutes *severe*—simply because they have never seen and worked with "severely" depressed patients. Nonprofessionals, of course, usually have even less experience with the range of normal and abnormal moods. Without the experience of seeing and treating many patients with depressive illnesses, it is impossible to accurately separate normal from abnormal mental experiences or "clinically significant" mood changes from those that are within the range of normal. In psychiatry as perhaps in no other field, the dictum "a little knowledge is a dangerous thing" holds true.

Second, many *medical* conditions can mimic abnormal mood states, dozens of pharmaceuticals can cause depression or euphoric states in some persons, and drugs of abuse can cause all kinds of mood states and psychoses in almost anyone. Almost all the DSM diagnoses contain "exclusion criteria" for medical conditions, such as "the symptoms are not due to . . . a general medical condition." Only a clinician trained in the diagnosis and treatment of physical illness will be able to pick up these sorts of problems.

Lastly, just as the range of normal experience and behavior is enormous, so is the range and complexity of abnormal mental experiences and behaviors—they cannot be contained in any one book and certainly not all described in a few dozen diagnostic categories.

For these reasons, I am not going to list the DSM diagnostic criteria for the disorders described in this chapter. I don't want to tempt nonclinicians to engage in self-diagnosis or diagnosis of family members. Also, the DSM is easily available in libraries—but it should be considered a reference book for clinicians, not a textbook of psychiatry.

A "MULTIAXIAL" DIAGNOSTIC SYSTEM

A formal DSM diagnosis always lists five types of diagnoses and other pieces of clinical information on patients in five separate categories, each of which is called an "axis."

Axis I	Clinical disorders
Axis II	Personality and intelligence
Axis III	General medical conditions
Axis IV	Psychosocial and environmental problems
Axis V	Assessment of level of functioning

The reason for this complexity is that, to put it plainly, people are complex creatures, and an understanding of their mental life requires looking at them from several different angles.

On *axis I* is listed the psychiatric illness or condition that is being treated or studied. This is where a mood disorder diagnosis would go, as would diagnoses such as attention-deficit/hyperactivity disorder or panic disorder or alcohol abuse. This diagnosis often includes additional descriptive terms such as *chronic, acute, severe,* or *recurrent.*

Because symptoms of a psychiatric illness might be expressed differently depending on a person's personality and intellectual ability, these two factors are also recorded for every patient—on *axis II.* Because these factors affect how a person copes with a particular psychiatric illness, they are very important in developing plans for treating the disorder. This is also where a diagnosis of a *personality disorder* goes. A personality disorder is diagnosed when the patient's personality—a complex mix of temperament, attitudes and habits, ways of approaching life's problems, attitudes towards self and others—causes problems in relationships and functioning.

A person with "avoidant personality disorder," for example, is socially inhibited, hypersensitive to negative comments or reactions from others, and constantly fearful of criticism and rejection. These individuals are so sensitized to criticism that they see it everywhere and avoid making friends or even going to social activities. They withdraw from life and function below their true capabilities because of these fears and preoccupations. This pattern of thinking, relating, and behaving is called a personality disorder because it seems ingrained in the individual's personality from an early age rather than the expression of an illness imposed upon him or her at some point in life.

Personality disorder diagnoses are not made very often in adolescents, for several reasons. The most important one is that in young persons, personality style is still under development. Personality traits that are present in childhood often do not persist into adult life. Another reason is that prolonged periods of depression can negatively affect adolescents' ways of thinking about themselves and their relationships. You've already seen how depression can adversely affect how young persons relate to others and color their view of themselves and their world. It's not difficult, then, to see how a chronically depressed young person can seem to have the personality style and show the behaviors of avoidant personality disorder briefly described above, and thus seem to meet the criteria for this diagnosis. But to make a diagnosis of a personality disorder would be to miss the most important problem: depression. Technically, a diagnosis of personality disorder can be made in someone under the age of 18 if the personality traits have been present and causing problems for at least one year. Nevertheless, for the reasons I've mentioned, most psychiatrists are reluctant (or at least they should be) to make a personality disorder diagnosis in an adolescent, especially an adolescent who is or has been depressed.

Also listed on axis II is a diagnosis of mental retardation.

Axis III is the place to list any medical problem the individual may have. Examples would be high blood pressure, asthma, kidney failure, or migraine headaches. The axis III diagnosis is sometimes very important in treating a patient with a mood disorder, because mood symptoms can be caused or affected by medical conditions such as thyroid problems or medications being taken for a medical problem. Medication that an adolescent might be taking for asthma, for example, can cause nervousness and anxiety.

On *axis IV* are listed problems in and stresses from the environment that may contribute to the patient's difficulties—parental divorce, serious illness in the adolescent or another family member, a move to a new community, chronic poverty, living in an unsafe neighborhood. These factors can also affect how individuals cope with illness as well as their response to treatment. Axis IV information is especially important in the mood disorders, since environmental stressors can be an important precipitating factor for an episode of illness.

On *axis V*, the clinician records an assessment of the patient's functional level, using a 1 to 100 rating scale called the Global Assessment of Functioning (GAF) Scale. This assessment is a judgment of how impaired (or unimpaired) a patient is by symptoms in everyday life. On this scale, a score of 80 or above indicates basically normal everyday functioning, below 50 indicates serious impairment such as recurrent unemployment due to psychiatric illness, and below 20 indicates a level of impairment that suggests the need for psychiatric hospitalization. This axis is perhaps more useful to researchers and statisticians than to clinicians, but it serves to round out a picture of the patient, capturing strengths as opposed to afflictions. For example, an individual might suffer from a severe psychiatric disorder such as schizophrenia, have a low IQ, suffer from diabetes, and live at the poverty level, but, despite all these handicaps, be a good parent who contributes to her community—an axis V rating would indicate that despite her psychiatric, intellectual, medical, and environmental problems, this person is functioning rather well. This hypothetical patient's DSM IV diagnoses would be as follows:

Axis I	Schizophrenia, paranoid type
Axis II	Mild mental retardation
Axis III	Diabetes
Axis IV	Poverty
Axis V	GAF = 80

MOOD DISORDER CATEGORIES IN DSM IV

I've already discussed the two main depressive disorder categories: major depressive disorder and dysthymic disorder. *Major depressive disorder* is the most frequently diagnosed depressive disorder of adolescence. It is characterized by one or more major depressive episodes and periods of recovery between episodes. *Dysthymic disorder* is the smoldering disorder in which symptoms persist for months at a time. According to the DSM, symptoms must persist for at least one year in children and adolescents. (Adults must show symptoms for two years.)

Serious depressive illnesses that don't quite fit the diagnostic criteria for either of these disorders are called in the DSM *depressive disorder not otherwise specified* (*depressive disorder NOS*). This is something of a "wastebasket" category and a good example of why the DSM should not be considered a psychiatric "bible" when it comes to understanding and treating patients. An adolescent who has had symptoms of dysthymic disorder for 364 days would technically need to be diagnosed with depressive disorder NOS until, on the 365th day, the diagnosis could be changed to dysthymic disorder—obviously not a very meaningful distinction for an individual patient. People with severe depression who don't have enough symptoms on a DSM checklist also technically need to be put into this category. The DSM should be seen as a guide to diagnosis and treatment, not a textbook. It would be wise to repeat my favorite quote from Alfred Kinsey here: "The world is not divided into sheep and goats . . . Nature rarely deals with discrete categories. Only the human mind invents categories and tries to force facts into separated pigeonholes."[2] I've already discussed some of the difficulties in separating depressive disorders in young persons into discrete categories and some of the problems with symptom overlap. Mood disorders often can't be divided simply into this category or that one—and individuals often don't fit into DSM pigeonholes.

The symptoms and the course of illness of two subtypes of bipolar disorder have been sufficiently well characterized to get their own DSM categories, *bipolar I* and *bipolar II*. As we saw in chapter 3, there are probably other forms of bipolar illness that will eventually be described and understood well enough to be demarcated with their own label, but for now a patient having another of these "soft" bipolar disorders would be diagnosed with *bipolar disorder not otherwise specified* (*bipolar disorder* NOS), according to the DSM. *Cyclothymic disorder* is also included in the DSM IV as an axis I diagnosis.

For people with bipolar I disorder, the clinician, when using the DSM, is supposed to specify the type of the patient's latest episode, as in *bipolar I disorder, most recent episode manic*, or *bipolar I disorder, most recent episode depressed*.

The DSM also provides several other descriptive terms, called *specifiers*, that can be added to the main diagnosis to better describe the current episode of mood problems. The clinician can call the episode *mild, moderate*, or *severe*. If the patient has not had any episodes in two months, the disorder can be designated *in remission* (*in full remission* if there have been no symptoms for two months, *in partial remission* if only a few symptoms or the remission has been less than two months). If the patient has all the symptoms of major depression continuously for a period of at least two years, major depression is said to be *chronic*.

The specifier *with melancholic features* can be added when the patient's depressive episode is dominated by loss of ability to experience pleasure (anhedonia) and by guilty feelings, loss of appetite, and the classic daily fluctuation of mood (early morning awakening, with the mood lifting slightly as the day progresses)—in short, the "textbook" depressive syndrome so eloquently described by William Styron in *Darkness Visible*.

Another clinical syndrome (more common in depressive disorders than in bipolar disorders) has been called *atypical depression*. People with this syndrome retain reactivity in their mood (their mood brightens when good things happen), in fact, they seem to have a "hyper-reactive" mood and an especially difficult time with rejection in interpersonal relationships—even when not in an episode of depression. They also tend to have changes in appetite and sleep of the less common pattern: eating and sleeping too much. This syndrome was considered very rare in young people for many years, but an article in the *Journal of the American Academy of Child and Adolescent Psychiatry* in 2000 indicates that it may not be so uncommon after all. These clinicians found that more than 15 percent of the depressed children and youths they interviewed met the diagnostic criteria for atypical depression. They also cautioned, however, that the symptoms often didn't hang together very well: many patients didn't have all or even most of the symptoms.[3]

If the mood episode occurs within four week of the birth of a child, it is called *with postpartum onset*. For dysthymic disorder, the specifiers *early onset* (before age 21) or *late onset* (after age 21) may be used.

The specifier *with psychotic features* can be added if the patient has hallucinations or delusional beliefs during the illness, such as those described in chapter 2. The specifier *with catatonic features* is added if the patient shows symptoms of catatonia, a rare syndrome in which the individual lies (or sometime sits or stands) motionless for long periods of time staring into space and has other unusual physical mannerisms such as rigid posturing, grimacing, or meaninglessly repeating whatever is said to him or her. Both of these problems are unusual in adolescent depressions.

Another set of specifiers describes the course of the illness over time, called *longitudinal course specifiers*. Mood disorders may be *with* or *without full inter-episode recovery*, depending on whether the individual is completely free of symptoms between episodes or not.

Some people have a mood disorder in which they have repeated depressive episodes occurring regularly in the winter and sometimes hypomanic or manic symptoms in the summer. This illness has been called "seasonal affective disorder." In DSM IV, the specifier *with seasonal pattern* is added to the diagnosis of major depressive or bipolar disorder.

Lastly, patients with a bipolar disorder who have had at least four episodes in twelve months have a disorder *with rapid cycling*.

When drug intoxication or medical problems mimic depressive episodes, the DSM diagnoses *substance-induced mood disorder* or *mood disorder due to a general medical condition* are used. When the mood problem is due to a medical condition, the medical condition and type of mood

Table 4-1 Mood Disorders in the DSM

Major Depressive Disorder

Full syndrome of severe depression

    Severity specifiers

        —mild, moderate, severe (with or without psychotic features)

        —in partial or full remission

    Special syndrome specifiers

        —with melancholic, catatonic, or atypical features

        —with postpartum onset

    Longitudinal course specifiers

        —with or without full inter-episode recovery

        —with seasonal pattern

        —chronic

Dysthymic Disorder

Smoldering, low-grade, long-standing depression

        —early onset (before age 21)

        —late onset (after age 21)

        —with atypical features

Depressive Disorder NOS

Bipolar Disorder I

Mania and severe depression

Bipolar Disorder II

Severe depression and hypomania

    Specifiers for bipolar disorders:

    Severity specifiers

        —mild, moderate, severe (with or without psychotic features)

        —in partial or full remission

    Special syndrome specifiers

        —with melancholic, catatonic, or atypical features

        —with postpartum onset

    Longitudinal course specifiers

        —with or without full inter-episode recovery

        —with seasonal pattern

        —with rapid cycling

Bipolar Disorder NOS

"Soft" bipolar and bipolar spectrum disorders

Cyclothymic Disorder

Depressive symptoms and hypomanias

Substance-Induced Mood Disorder

Mood Disorder Due to a General Medical Condition

change are specified in the diagnosis (as in, for example, "mood disorder due to hyperthyroidism, with manic features"). When the problem is due to substance abuse, the type of mood change and whether the symptoms came on during intoxication or withdrawal are specified. (Examples would be "alcohol-induced mood disorder with depressive features, onset during withdrawal" and "cocaine-induced mood disorder with manic features, onset during intoxication.")

CONTROVERSIES IN THE USE OF THE DSM

There have been enormous controversies surrounding the use of the DSM in the diagnosis of psychiatric problems in children and adolescents. Although these controversies don't touch very directly on the use of DSM diagnoses for mood disorders, a brief discussion is still warranted. The misuse of psychiatric diagnosis is, and should be, an important concern for parents.

The problems with the DSM arise with the various diagnoses that get applied to children and adolescents with behavioral problems: problems involving high activity levels, defiant behaviors, and disruptive and destructive behaviors. The main criticism usually leveled at the DSM is that it "medicalizes" problems in children that are really no more than normal behavioral and developmental variations of one type or another. The parents of a child who is more energetic and less attentive than his classmates get a letter from the teacher recommending that the child be evaluated for attention deficit disorder. When does "inattention" become attention deficit disorder? How does anyone decide what constitutes a "disorder"?

In earlier chapters I made the point that most of the problems psychiatrists are called on to treat do not have any known physical basis—no abnormalities on brain scans or blood tests (what are called *biological markers* for psychiatric illness). This means that the diagnostic criteria are basically things that the person experiences or does: thoughts, feelings, and behaviors. A problem arises when what are identified as "symptoms" are experiences or behaviors that are not outside the realm of normal, except as to degree.

There is little disagreement that hearing voices when no one is speaking is not normal. And the frenzied disorganization of mania can't be mistaken for normal high spirits. But what about a childhood diagnosis such as *conduct disorder*, for which the symptoms are behaviors like fighting, setting fires, disobedience, and running away? How does one decide when "bad behavior" becomes "*really* bad behavior," then becomes conduct disorder? Even more slippery is *oppositional defiant disorder*, for which the diagnostic criteria include things like "often loses temper," "often argues with adults," "is often angry and resentful," and "is often touchy or easily annoyed by others." An adolescent who has had these characteristics for six months to the point where they cause "clinically significant impairment" in her school or family life would meet the DSM criteria for this diagnosis. Now, from what you already know about depression, you can see that a depressed adolescent may be all of these things. Does Heather in the vignette in chapter 3 have both major depressive disorder *and* oppositional defiant disorder? Although, technically, she does not, because the DSM diagnosis of oppositional defiant disorder cannot be made when the symptoms occur during an episode of depression, you can see how complicated and difficult the issue of psychiatric diagnosis can sometimes be. For every voice calling for the early identification and treatment of psychiatric problems in young people, there seems to be another one warning that overdiagnosing and, worse, overmedicating young people is the real problem, and a more sinister one at that.

How are these controversies important for the parent of a depressed adolescent? First and foremost, they reinforce what I have been saying about the DSM being only a guide to psychiatric diagnosis—and a decidedly imperfect one. Second, they should make parents cautious and questioning about the diagnosis of a behavioral disorder in their child if they notice signs of depression. Using the DSM criteria for behavioral disorders as a checklist to assess difficult behaviors so as to assign diagnoses such as conduct disorder and oppositional defiant disorder, while missing a depression or other causes of these clusters of behaviors, happens all too frequently—especially when the DSM is in the hands of persons without much training in the assessment of psychiatric illnesses. Third, and perhaps most important, parents should be skeptical of some people's insistence on the opposite view: that the behavioral symptoms of serious depressive illnesses are no more than "bad behavior" and, worse, that punishment rather than treatment is necessary to teach adolescents about the "consequences" of their bad behaviors.

Unlike some other DSM categories, depressive disorders in adolescence have a clear demarcation from normal behaviors and need medical treatment. That treatment is the subject of the next part of the book.

PART II

Treatment

In these chapters, I discuss the available treatments for adolescent depression. We now have a wide range of treatments, from pharmaceutical and other medical treatments to specific types of psychotherapy that have proved especially helpful in treating depression.

Chapter 5 introduces some of the special considerations that must be given to the use of medications in the adolescent age range. After all, some adolescents are physically more like children, whereas others are close to adults. Are medications given in different dosages to adolescents? Are the medications known to be effective in treating adult depression also effective in adolescents? These are some of the questions answered here. I also present a brief introduction to what we know about the chemical workings of the brain and how the medications used to treat depression work.

In chapters 6 through 8, I talk more specifically about medical treatment, reviewing the various pharmaceuticals used to treat these illnesses. In chapter 8, I include some less frequently used medications, an herbal treatment for depression, and electroconvulsive therapy—still a very valuable resource for the treatment of mood disorders. This chapter ends with a discussion of several promising experimental treatments for severe depression. Finally, chapter 9 covers the role of counseling and psychotherapy in treating youngsters with depression.

CHAPTER 5

Medication Issues in Adolescence

We know that the medications used to treat adult disorders don't always work in quite the same way in children and adolescents. Unfortunately, textbooks, research articles, and prescribing guidelines from pharmaceutical manufacturers often provide only limited guidance about the use of medications to treat psychiatric problems in children and adolescents. One reason for this is that far fewer good research studies have been conducted on the use of psychiatric medications in these younger patients than on their use in adults. Pharmaceutical research is more difficult to do in young people, for a variety of reasons. Parents who would themselves willingly volunteer to be in a drug study are often much less willing to volunteer their children for research, making it difficult to recruit research subjects. Issues of informed consent to be a research subject are much more complicated when minors are involved, making researchers reluctant to tackle the issue. Not only are these studies more challenging to do, but the financial returns for pharmaceutical companies are often far lower: children and adolescents usually represent a smaller "market" for medications than do adults.

These factors have added up to a lack of information about the use of psychiatric medications in children and adolescents compared with that available for prescribing to adults. The prescription of psychiatric medication to young people is often what is referred to as "off-label" prescribing, a term I'll explain below.

PHARMACEUTICALS AND THE FDA

The United States Food and Drug Administration (FDA) is responsible for determining that a pharmaceutical is safe for use in humans and that it is effective for the illness or symptoms for which the manufacturer claims it is effective. The FDA's process of determining the safety of pharmaceuticals is quite thorough, perhaps the most thorough and rigorous in the world. It is credited with preventing an epidemic in the United States of birth defects caused by thalidomide, which occurred in other countries during the 1960s. Thalidomide was widely used in Europe but had not been approved for sale in the United States when it was discovered to cause severe deforming birth defects in children whose mothers had taken it during pregnancy.

A pharmaceutical company performs, sponsors, and encourages research on a drug it wants to sell and then presents the research results to the FDA in support of its request to sell the drug and market it to physicians. Once the drug is approved, the product can be sold in the United States and the FDA regulates how the drug is "labeled" for use. This "labeling" is the information on the product insert distributed with the drug to physicians and patients. The FDA does not regulate how physicians can prescribe a given pharmaceutical. A doctor can legally prescribe an approved drug for *any* purpose she wants to, based on her knowledge of the medical research literature and using her medical judgment—even if the FDA has not reviewed the effectiveness of the drug for that particular use. When a doctor prescribes a pharmaceutical for an illness or symptom that is not covered in the drug's labeling, this is called *off-label* prescribing. The FDA also strictly regulates how a drug is advertised and marketed to physicians by representatives of the pharmaceutical companies.

There are a number of reasons that physicians quite frequently prescribe pharmaceuticals for off-label indications. Once a drug has been approved for sale, manufacturers often are very conservative about requesting the FDA to approve a new use for the drug (called the drug's *indication*), even if clinical research shows the new use is an effective one. For example, research had shown quite clearly that antidepressant medications were effective in the treatment of panic attacks for many years before the FDA labeled any antidepressants for treating panic disorder; many antidepressants are still not labeled for this use but are widely and safely prescribed for panic attacks. Research had shown that the antiepilepsy medication divalproex was a safe and effective treatment for manic symptoms for many years before its manufacturer, Abbott Laboratories, requested that its brand of divalproex, Depakote, be approved to treat mania. Off-label prescription of a pharmaceutical for a particular condition often precedes "FDA-approved" prescribing for that condition by years, even decades. As of this writing, the antidepressant sertraline (Zoloft) is labeled for the treatment of obsessive-compulsive disorder in children 6 to 17 years old but not for the treatment of depression, even though more prescriptions are probably written for the treatment of depression than for obsessive-compulsive disorder in this age range.

A pharmaceutical company's sales representatives are not permitted to discuss off-label uses of their company's products when they make marketing visits to physicians, but, as I've noted, the drug can be prescribed for any purpose that the physician thinks will safely help her patient.

What are the reasons for these inconsistencies and delays? There are several. Perhaps the most important is that once a medication has been approved for one indication, a pharmaceutical manufacturer may decide that it's not particularly advantageous to request a new indication, especially if the new indication is for a less common condition. The expense of going through an FDA approval process may not be offset by the increase in sales that marketing the drug for the new indication would bring about—especially since doctors are able to prescribe the medication off-label anyway. This means that the labeling of any pharmaceutical is usually an incomplete guide to the use of a medication and illustrates why a physician must have a familiarity with the clinical research literature to make prescribing decisions. The popular *Physicians' Desk Reference* (the PDR) is *not* a good source of information about medications and prescribing, for this very reason: the PDR is only a compilation of the FDA labeling for medications. If physicians limited themselves to only FDA-approved uses of pharmaceuticals, many patients would go untreated for conditions for which proven remedies are available.

Just as a pharmaceutical company may decide it's not financially advantageous to ask the FDA to label a drug for a new indication, the company may decide there are no financial incentives to ask the FDA to label a drug for prescription to children and adolescents. If you glance through the PDR, you'll notice that for many medications, it makes no mention of uses in children and adolescents and gives only the recommended doses in adults. Many psychiatric medications fall into this category. The FDA is addressing this vacuum, and policy revisions are in the works with new requirements to address the use of medications in young people when approval is sought for new pharmaceuticals.

DOSE ADJUSTMENTS AND OTHER DIFFERENCES FOR YOUNG PEOPLE

The dosing of medications is more complicated for young people than for adults. On the one hand, because children are physically smaller than adults, pediatric doses of medication are often smaller than adult doses. But then again, a healthy 16-year-old who is mature for his age may be physically bigger than many adults and require a dose of medication in the adult range, perhaps even at the top of the adult range. Sometimes a dosing guide is available that calls for a calculation of the appropriate dose of a medication based on body weight—but physical size differences between children and adults are only a part of the story. Many medications are absorbed into fat tissue, and at various ages young people and adults have different proportions of fatty tissue. This factor can be especially important in adolescents, because the distribution of fat tissue can change dramatically during puberty over a short period of time, especially in girls, requiring more frequent dosage adjustments than in adults.

Young people sometimes absorb medications from the gastrointestinal tract into their bloodstream more rapidly than do adults. This means that after a dose of medication, the level of medication in the blood rises more rapidly and to a higher peak level in youngsters than in adults. This can cause more sleepiness or other side effects immediately after taking the medication. Splitting the dose of medication into several doses throughout the day may help with this problem, but also means there are twice or even three times as many opportunities to forget to take a dose.

Young people and adults also eliminate medications differently. The amount of medication active in the body is determined by a balance between how much is going in and how much is going out: the main organ in charge of the "going out" part is the liver, which chemically breaks down most medications into inactive forms, which are then usually eliminated through the kidneys into the urine. In children, the liver is larger in proportion to overall body size than it is in adults. This means that children may eliminate a medication more quickly and may therefore need a surprisingly higher dose than would be expected from their physical stature.

All these differences decrease, of course, as a young person grows from child to adolescent to young adult. But remember that the timing of these physical changes can vary quite a bit from one individual to another. One particular 15-year-old might need to take a pediatric dose of a medication, while another might require an adult dose, because of these differences in physical maturity.

In addition to dosing differences, there may be important efficacy differences between young people and adults. That is, just because a medication is effective in adults for a particular problem doesn't mean it will be equally effective for what seems to be a similar problem in a child or adolescent. The most striking example of this is the difference in efficacy of certain antidepressants. The class of antidepressants called tricyclic antidepressants has been used with great effectiveness to treat depressive disorders in adults for many years, and it was assumed that tricyclics must be effective in childhood depression as well. But in a number of clinical studies done in the 1980s, tricyclics appeared no more effective than placebo (a "sugar pill") in treating childhood depression. (Other types of studies do show some efficacy; I discuss this controversy in the next chapter.) It may be that the different symptoms often seen in younger depression patients are a reflection of differences in the chemical basis of their depression, or perhaps a difference between the developing nervous system and the mature brain makes younger patients respond to some medications differently.

All of these issues mean that the dosing rules and guidelines for prescribing most psychiatric medications for young people are still developing. A glance through the PDR *is not* a good way to get information about medications. A discussion with the prescribing physician about his reasoning in picking a particular dose of medication *is*.

HOW PSYCHIATRIC MEDICATIONS WORK

A number of years ago, psychiatrist and neuroscientist Nancy Andreason wrote the book *The Broken Brain*, about the new discoveries in biological psychiatry.[1] The title makes the point that psychiatric illnesses such as major depressive disorder, bipolar disorder, and schizophrenia are caused by biological and chemical malfunctions of the brain, not repressed memories or traumatic childhoods. Although we still don't know exactly what these malfunctions are, we are getting very close to understanding some of the biological mechanisms that might be involved in the symptoms of mood disorders.

In order to understand the treatment of mood disorders with medications, you should know a little bit about how the brain works. Patients and parents frequently ask, "What does this medication *do?*" The answer to this question turns out to be complicated, so, in this chapter, I'm going to give a brief overview of the functioning of the human nervous system, just enough to help you understand a little bit about how psychiatric medications work.

Many people imagine that the human brain is a kind of wonderful computer. Although this is a vast oversimplification of the true capabilities of the brain, it's a good place to start in trying to understand how this fantastic organ of the mind works.

Like the computer that I'm using to write these words, a human brain receives input, processes the information it receives, and then delivers output. Like a computer, it stores information and often uses this stored information to help process the input it receives. The brain receives its input from the sense organs—the eyes, ears, taste buds, touch receptors, and so forth—and delivers output in the form of behavior.

The simplest example of this input-processing-output circuit in our nervous system is the spinal reflex. This circuit is so simple and so automatic in its operation that it richly deserves its label, *reflex*, meaning a simple behavior that requires no "thinking" to be effectively carried out. If you inadvertently touch the hot surface of a stove or a candle flame, a nerve ending detects the resulting tissue damage and fires a message along a nerve fiber (a sensory nerve) that ends in the spinal cord. Here, the first nerve communicates with another nerve, which dispatches a message down again through another fiber (a motor nerve) to activate the arm muscles to pull the finger back from the source of heat. If you've ever actually had this experience, you may have noticed that your hand pulled away before you even felt the pain. This is because the brain, where consciousness resides, is not yet involved. (The message that is eventually sent up to the brain from the level of the spinal cord responding to the pain signal is more or less a "FYI" message that will be stored in the memory system. Hopefully, this painful memory will lessen the chances of the same thing happening again.)

Let's look at a more complicated example of the input-processing-output circuit—one that is more than a reflex. Say you're walking down the

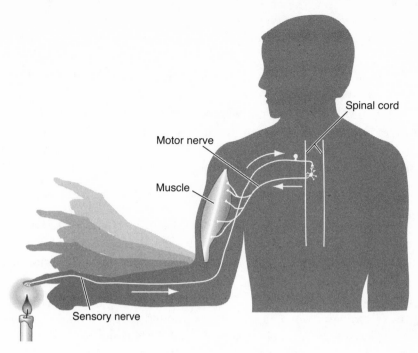

Figure 5-1 Spinal reflex

street and pass a florist shop with a sign in the window that reads, "Don't forget, next Sunday is Mother's Day!" You realize with a start that you *have* forgotten, so you go into the shop, pull out your credit card, and order some flowers. This is not really so different a process from the spinal reflex: input (seeing the sign), processing (I forgot!), and output (ordering the flowers). There are a lot more steps (and some very complex ones) this time around: seeing the sign, using the language functions of the brain to draw meaning from all those little shapes we call letters, drawing on memories of what is expected of you on Mother's Day, an emotional tone generated by your feelings for your mother that affects the process—just to name a few. A complex interaction of many, many nervous system functions is going on, some fairly simple (the posture reflexes that let you walk into the shop without falling are nearly as simple as the spinal reflex example above) and others more complex (the arithmetic functions that allow you to answer the question, "How big an arrangement can I buy without going over my credit limit?"). The processes are so complex, in fact, that no computer built today is capable of anything approaching as complex a processing task as this.

You may know that a computer computes by means of many thousands of microscopic switches embedded into its processing chip. The pattern of "on" and "off" in the switches is what stores information, and the flow of input signal through these switches is the processing. The human brain contains about eleven billion nerve cells, or neurons, but as powerful as a computer with eleven billion switches might be, our brain is much more impressive than that. The neuron is not simply a switch that is either "on" or "off"; rather, it is an impressive microprocessor in its own right. Each neuron receives input from many other neurons, processes this information, and sends output to many others. The brain is not simply a biological computer with billions of switches. It is more like a network of billions of computers, each capable of being individually programmed. Every neuron in the brain may receive input and transmit signals to up to fifty thousand other neurons. This makes the number of *all* the possible connections between neurons in the human brain incomprehensibly huge, a hyperastronomical number on the order of the number of molecules in the universe. (Even if we could figure out how to build such a computer, there'd be no place on the planet big enough to put it.) This almost unimaginable complexity explains why the capabilities of even the most powerful computers are puny compared with those of the human brain.

Like computers, the human nervous system uses electrical signals to do much of its work, as well as *chemical* signals called *neurotransmitters*.

Let's go back for a moment to the spinal reflex to examine how these signals do their jobs. Remember that in this reflex, a pain signal from the finger travels up a nerve fiber into the spinal cord. As you might guess, this is an electrical signal, a change in the electrical charge of the nerve fiber that travels as a pulse along the length of the fiber until it reaches a "cell body" that resides in the spinal cord. This cell body is one of the eleven billion tiny computers I mentioned earlier (except that it's in the spinal cord, not in the brain). When a sufficient number of pain signals arrive at the cell body, this microscopic CPU starts communicating with the motor nerve responsible for pulling away the finger, and when the motor neuron computes that it's necessary, this neuron fires its own pulse of electrical energy down the motor nerve to the muscles. The signals by which the neurons communicate with each other are the chemical ones I mentioned above: molecules called neurotransmitters. Most of the medications used in psychiatry work by affecting neurotransmitters in one way or another.

One neuron sends a chemical signal to another at a site called the *synapse,* an area where the two neurons nearly touch, separated only by an ultramicroscopic space called the *synaptic cleft.* The first neuron (the *presynaptic neuron*) releases packets of neurotransmitters that flow across the narrow synaptic cleft and link up with targets called *receptors* on the next cell (the *postsynaptic neuron*); the neurotransmitter molecules fit into their receptors like keys fit into locks. There needs to be some mechanism for this signaling system to be turned off and reset, of course. After neurotransmitter molecules in one pulse link up with receptors across the synapse, they must somehow be removed in preparation for the next pulse. This happens in a variety of ways in different cells, but one of the most important mechanisms is *reuptake* into the cell that released them. A reuptake pump on the presynaptic neuron removes neurotransmitter molecules from the synapse and takes them into the interior of the cell, where they are repackaged for re-release.

There is a constant level of neurotransmitter release across the synapse, a steady tone of chemical signal that pulses up at times. The neurons are not just "switches" that can only be set to "on" or "off" but rather tiny information-processing units that are constantly communicating with other neurons to which they are functionally linked.

Now let's return to mood disorders. What is "broken" in these illnesses? As you will see, much of what we know about the biological and chemical basis of mood disorders was discovered *after* an effective medication had been accidentally discovered. In a backwards kind of investigative process, by figuring out where in the brain these medications are active and what they do to brain chemistry (usually by observing the effects of these pharmaceuticals on brain preparations in test tubes), we have found clues about the location and function of the "broken" mechanisms in mood disorders.

In chapter 1, I mentioned that the first pharmaceutical to have antidepressant effects, iproniazid, was discovered accidentally when doctors noticed that depressed tuberculosis patients taking the drug for their lung disease had improvement in their mood symptoms. In 1957, another breakthrough in the treatment of mood disorders occurred when Roland Kuhn, a Swiss psychiatrist, discovered that a compound originally developed as an antihistamine also had remarkable therapeutic effects on depressed patients. He reported his results in a Swiss medical journal, in a paper titled "The Treatment of Depressive States with G 22355 (Imipramine Hydrochloride)."[2] Unlike iproniazid, imipramine is still used as an antidepressant medication.

Figure 5-2 Synapse

For many years, brain scientists had only vague ideas about the answer to the question, "What does imipramine *do*?" When some of them started to look at the effect of this pharmaceutical on brain chemistry, they discovered that imipramine was a powerful inhibitor of the reuptake of a group of neurotransmitters called *neurogenic amines*, or *neuroamines*, the most important of these being *norepinephrine*.

Remember that neurons turn off their chemical signals (turn *down* is probably more accurate) by scooping up neurotransmitter molecules from the synapse and repackaging them. Just as partially closing the drain in a bathtub while the water is running will cause the tub to begin to fill with water, blocking the reuptake of neurotransmitter molecules has the net effect of *increasing* neurotransmitters in the synapse. This observation, that antidepressants increase the amount of neurotransmitters in the synapse by blocking their reuptake, led to the "amine hypothesis" of the mood disorders. This hypothesis basically stated that an abnormally low level of norepinephrine caused depression and that, in bipolar disorder, too high a level caused mania.

Further work soon indicated that this explanation was too simplistic. As more antidepressant medications were discovered, it was found that some very effective ones seemed to have little effect on the norepinephrine system. Fluoxetine (Prozac) is one of a family of pharmaceuticals that are powerful inhibitors of the reuptake of another neurotransmitter, called *serotonin*, but they have very little direct effect on norepinephrine. Some antidepressants also seem to affect other neurotransmitters too, especially one called *dopamine*. As a result of these discoveries, the amine hypothesis was revised and the proposal was put forward that mood is regulated by a complex interplay of *several* chemical circuits in the brain. It is now thought that the interplay of activity among *all* these systems is disrupted in depression and in mania.

Another argument against a simplistic theory involving too much or too little norepinephrine is an observation about the time course of the antidepressant-induced chemical changes in the brain. Antidepressant-induced changes in neurotransmitter levels at the synapse occur almost *immediately* after the drug is taken—in a matter of hours. But, as is well known, several *weeks* are required for these agents to start alleviating the symptoms of depression. If the problem were simply too little neurotransmitter in the synapses of certain brain circuits, why would it take several *weeks* after the drug raised transmitter levels at the synapse for the symptoms of depression to get better? It has been suggested that the neurons respond to these higher levels of neurotransmitters by changing their receptor molecules, either making them more sensitive to the neurotransmitter or putting more of them on the surface of the postsynaptic cell. The idea is that antidepressants work by triggering an "up-regulation" of receptor sensitivity in the neuron. This hypothesis continues to be popular among neuroscientists interested in the chemistry of mood disorders.

This idea fits nicely with some of the work done on the chemical mapping of the brain. Several nuclei of cells (*nucleus* here means a group of neurons) deep in the brain that use norepinephrine as their neurotransmitter project a vast network of fibers that terminate on sheets of cells contained on the convoluted surface of the brain, the cerebral cortex. The cerebral cortex, thought to be responsible for many of our most complex "higher" brain functions, is rich in cells with receptors for norepinephrine. This system seems to be ideally organized to affect the tone of functioning of the entire cerebral cortex—making it a good candidate for the target system of antidepressants. There are serotonin pathways that originate deep in the brain and project widely across the cortex too, as well as pathways that use other neurotransmitters. The balance of activity among these different systems and their interaction with each other are probably very important in the regulation of mood. These neurotransmitter systems are most likely the sites where antidepressant medications do their work.

Because of the uniquely therapeutic effects of *lithium* in bipolar disorder and its important antidepressant effects, a lot of effort has gone into trying to figure out the site of lithium's activity in the brain and its effect on brain chemistry. Lithium doesn't seem to affect neuroamine levels anything like antidepressants do, and it doesn't interact with neuroamine receptors or the reuptake pumps. In fact, it doesn't have any of the types of direct effects on cells that the antidepressants have. Only in the last few years has the probable site of lithium action been found, and it's not at the synapse at all. Lithium (and perhaps the newer mood stabilizers as well) seems to work at a different cellular level: *inside* the neuron.

Although the precise fit between a neurotransmitter and its receptor molecule has often been compared to the precise fit of a key into a lock, it has become apparent that the receptor is much more than just a lock. Starting in the 1970s, scientists were able to elucidate the structure of cellular receptors and discover the details of these complex and elegant mechanisms. Receptors on the surface of the cell are coupled with structures called G *proteins*, which extend through the cell membrane (the outer covering of the cell) and link up with a complex array of other proteins and enzymes within the cell that help regulate various cellular functions. The G proteins act as transducers, converting data from outside the cell (the presence or

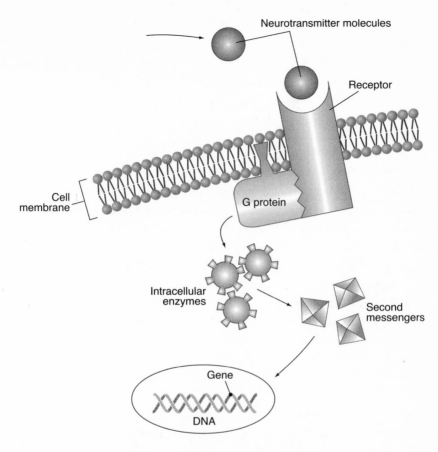

Figure 5-3 Receptors and G proteins

absence of neurotransmitters bound to the receptor molecules) into functional changes inside the cell. They don't do this directly but by a complex cascade of chemical events that probably also includes turning genes
inside the cell on and off.

There is evidence that lithium has direct effects on G proteins, but scientists have recently started to focus on several other groups of molecules
that work inside the cell as "second messengers." The neurotransmitters,
molecules that bring messages from other cells to the neuron, are considered the *first* messengers. The *second* messengers are molecules *inside* the
cell that are activated by G proteins to travel within the neuron to activate
various cellular switches in the cell membrane and in the cell nucleus, the
main control center of the neuron. Several lines of evidence support the

alternative idea that lithium acts by inhibiting enzymes responsible for the manufacture of several second messenger molecules.

One might think of the G protein–second messenger system as a communications and activity-monitoring system for the neuron, constantly assessing the level of neurotransmitter activity and, perhaps by turning genes on and off, constantly altering and adjusting the functioning of the neuron in response to this activity. This process might be a necessary part of maintaining mood within a normal range, and it might control mood by somehow "tuning" the responsiveness of our mood state to experiences and environment. Perhaps mood disorders are the result of a broken G protein–second messenger system in neurons of the norepinephrine and serotonin circuits that regulate mood: the system's sensitivity gets incorrectly tuned too high or too low and abnormal changes of mood result. (This might explain why the highs and lows of bipolar disorder are *both* effectively treated by lithium. Perhaps the lithium ion fits into and stabilizes the shape of one of the component molecules of this system or in some other way helps the system to work better and do its job more effectively, thus stabilizing mood.)

This idea may also explain why antidepressants take several weeks to work. Antidepressants may artificially raise neurotransmitter levels in the synapse to very high levels, high enough so that even a "broken" G protein–second messenger system can respond, turning on genes that start making receptor molecules or other cell components necessary to retune the neuron, a process that takes several weeks.

It may be a while before we understand how all the molecular and cellular pieces of this complicated story fit together, but the work to unravel the basic cause (or causes) of mood disorders is proceeding very rapidly. Adolescent patients and their parents frequently complain that they feel they are "guinea pigs" when it comes to picking medications to treat mood disorders, because there's really no way to know which medication or combination of medications will work best for a particular person. When we understand exactly what is "broken" in these illnesses, the job of treating them will become much easier and also much more systematic.

CHAPTER 6

Antidepressant Medications

Antidepressant medications have been used for several decades in treating children and adolescents, and the odds are that the first medication to be recommended for your child will be an antidepressant. These highly effective medications are safer than ever, and more and different antidepressants are being introduced every year.

Talking about this group of medications illustrates how the name of a class of medications often doesn't do them justice in describing their true range of efficacy. Medications listed as "antidepressants" have been found to be effective treatments for a whole variety of problems besides depression. In fact, more antidepressant prescriptions may be written to treat problems other than depression than to treat the illnesses for which these medications are named. Tricyclic antidepressants are effective in the treatment of panic attacks, obsessive-compulsive symptoms, and attention-deficit/hyperactivity disorder. Imipramine is effective in treating enuresis (bedwetting).

TRICYCLIC ANTIDEPRESSANTS

Although tricyclics are now prescribed less frequently than other, newer antidepressants, I start with this group because they were the first antidepressant medications developed and because they still provide the standard by which all promising new pharmaceuticals for the treatment of depression in adults are usually judged. As with most psychiatric medications, how-

CHCH₂CH₂N(CH₃)₂

$$CHCH_2CH_2N(CH_3)_2$$

AMITRIPTYLINE

$$CH_2CH_2CH_2N(CH_3)_2$$

IMIPRAMINE

Figure 6-1 Chemical structure of two tricyclic molecules, showing their characteristic three-ringed structure

ever, their use in adolescents for the treatment of depression has been mainly based on their proven effectiveness in adults, but recently some studies have thrown doubt on the assumption that they are just as effective in children and adolescents. These pharmaceuticals are called *tricyclics* because of the three rings in their chemical structure.

Although some of these medications have an effect on serotonin systems in the brain, the primary effect of the tricyclics seems to be an inhibition of reuptake of the neurotransmitter *norepinephrine* by neurons. Remember that reuptake of neurotransmitters into the neuron after they have been released into the synaptic cleft and done their work (signaling the next cell) is the means by which the synapse is "reset." Norepinephrine is usually quickly removed from the synapse and pumped back into the cell that released it, in order to turn off and reset the system. By blocking the removal of norepinephrine, tricyclics seem to prolong or intensify norepinephrine's message to the postsynaptic cell.

This effect of tricyclics on norepinephrine in neurons was one of the first chemical effects of a medication active in the brain to be measured in the laboratory. The observation that tricyclics *increased* the amount of norepinephrine in the synapse, along with the discovery that certain other medications used to treat high blood pressure *reduced* norepinephrine—and were observed to cause depression in some patients—led to the early

Table 6-1 Tricyclic Antidepressants

Generic Name	Brand Name
Amitriptyline	Elavil
Amoxapine	Asendin
Clomipramine	Anafranil
Desipramine	Norpramin
Doxepin	Sinequan
Imipramine	Tofranil
Maprotiline	Ludiomil
Nortriptyline	Pamelor
Protriptyline	Vivactil

"amine hypothesis" of the mood disorders: the theory that depression was caused by too little norepinephrine (and mania presumably by too much). However, further testing indicated that tricyclics increased amines in the synapse within *hours* of a person's taking them, whereas the therapeutic effects of antidepressants were known to take several *weeks*. This led to a search for alternatives to the amine hypothesis.

Following the discovery that tricyclics cause a change in the number and sensitivity of norepinephrine receptors on the postsynaptic neuron, it was suggested that this "down-regulation" of the norepinephrine system by tricyclics was the therapeutic effect of these medications for which researchers had been looking. But other, newer antidepressants don't have this down-regulating effect on norepinephrine.

The fundamental biochemical effect of antidepressants that is actually responsible for their benefits still remains a mystery. It is thought that the change in neuroamine signaling at the synapse caused by antidepressants may set off a cascade of events involving second messenger systems that eventually results in the improvement of the symptoms of depression. Unfortunately, how these medications work remains largely unknown. Imipramine, the tricyclic antidepressant first described by Roland Kuhn,[1] has been the most frequently prescribed medication of this type for young people.

The principal reason that tricyclics are now infrequently prescribed as antidepressant medications is their many side effects. As with all medications, some patients take these medications easily and without unpleasant side effects, but many have to put up with a few side effects in order to get the benefits. Fortunately, all the side effects are dose related and most are temporary.

You may remember that Dr. Kuhn found imipramine, the first tricyclic, among a group of compounds that had some antihistamine effects. It's not surprising, then, that these medications affect some people in the same way as antihistamines: causing mild sleepiness and sometimes what some of my patients have called a "weird" or "spacey" feeling for the first day or two after starting to take them. Tricyclics block another neurotransmitter, called acetylcholine, that is used in a division of the nervous system that regulates many "automatic" functions of the body, such as digestion. These *anticholinergic* side effects include a slowing down of the gastrointestinal tract, causing constipation and dry mouth. Focusing of the lens of the eye and emptying of the urinary bladder are also controlled by this system, and tricyclics can cause blurry vision and urination difficulties also, although usually only in high doses. Tricyclics also cause weight gain in many patients.

There have been several reports of sudden death in children taking desipramine, one of the tricyclic antidepressant medications, and a more recent sudden death in a child taking imipramine.[2] This appears to be an extremely rare event: less than half a dozen such cases have ever been reported. The cause has been presumed to be a sudden heart-rhythm problem, but this has never been proven. It has also been suggested that these were chance coincidences—that the deaths were not related to the medications. Nevertheless, many published guidelines recommend that, before starting to take a tricyclic antidepressant, children and adolescents have an electrocardiogram to make sure there is no undiagnosed heart problem.

Overdoses of tricyclics are very dangerous and are responsible for many of the completed suicides by overdose by people with mood disorders. For adults, the lethal overdose is up to twenty times the normal dose, but children are more sensitive to the toxic effects of these medications and just a handful of tablets can be fatal in a small child. For this reason, these medications must be scrupulously safeguarded in households with small children.

Accurate blood tests are available to measure tricyclic antidepressant levels in the bloodstream. The level at which these medications have their maximum efficacy, as well as ranges that are associated with side effects and toxicity, has been determined by clinical trials. These blood tests are very useful in adjusting the dosage of medication, especially if a usually adequate dose doesn't seem to be helping.

Children and adolescents eliminate these medications more quickly than do adults, perhaps because the size of the liver, the organ responsible for breaking down these medications, is proportionately larger in children than in adults. For this reason, monitoring of blood levels is especially important in adolescents to be sure they are getting the proper dose.

I've referred several times now to studies that have questioned the efficacy of these medications in treating depression in youngsters. There has been a discrepancy in results between what are referred to as "open" studies and "double-blind" studies of tricyclic medications in young people.

In an open study, the medication under investigation is given to a group of patients with the disorder for which the medication is thought to be effective, and the investigators simply assess how many patients get better and how many do not. Open studies have shown that between 60 and 80 percent of children have a therapeutic response to tricyclics, and significant recovery rates have been found in adolescents as well.[3]

There are two problems with open studies that can trick researchers into thinking a medication is effective when it really isn't. The biggest factor is the *placebo effect*. This is the beneficial effect that comes from taking a medication that is prescribed by a trusted source who is convinced of the effectiveness of the medication and who thus convinces the patient that the medication will help. When a person in a white coat writes a prescription or one in a white uniform gives you a pill, a powerful set of psychological factors is put into action that can make you feel significantly better. In an earlier chapter, I discussed the beneficial effect on demoralization of encouragement from a trusted source. It's easy to see, then, how the placebo effect can be especially powerful with antidepressant medications. The other factor that can mislead researchers in an open study is their own desire to get positive results: no matter how objective the researcher tries to be, there will always be a tendency, perhaps only an unconscious one, to accentuate the positive in measuring improvement in patients. Both these factors can lead to a finding in clinical trials of a medication benefit where there really isn't any.

Double-blind studies eliminate these misleading factors and are the most powerful type of medication trial possible—so much so that this type of study is now pretty much required for all new medications. In a double-blind placebo-controlled study, subjects who are similar in age, diagnosis, severity of illness, and so forth and who agree to be in the study are divided into two groups. One group (the *experimental* group) gets the medication that is being tested, and the other group (the *control* group) gets an identical-looking but inactive tablet, the placebo. The study participants do not know whether they are taking the new medication or the placebo, and neither do the clinicians who are examining them for improvement—hence the term *double*-blind. Only after the trial is over is the group membership of the participants revealed, and the results of the two groups are then compared. Improvement is measured objectively by using checklists of symptoms and various rating severity scales that have been verified as reliable and valid. (In some studies, instead of a placebo, the control group receives a standard medication for the disorder being studied. This allows researchers to study the use of new medications for serious illnesses for which it would be unethical to give patients a dummy pill and not have them receive available treatment for their condition. This type of study would be double-blind, but not placebo-controlled.)

Several double-blind placebo-controlled studies of tricyclic antidepressants in children and adolescents have shown no advantage of the drug over placebo.[4] Critics of these studies have argued that many of the subjects in the studies were only mildly depressed and were perhaps demoralized rather than suffering from a mood disorder, and thus were quite likely to have a placebo response. Some of the studies were of very small groups of patients and thus might not pick up the response for statistical reasons. Other studies have been criticized for not following up on the patients long enough to detect significant improvement and for using measures of improvement that were not sensitive enough.[5]

It seems reasonable to conclude that tricyclic antidepressants are not as effective in young people as they are in adults—though perhaps unreasonable to conclude that they are completely ineffective. This difference in efficacy has yet to be explained. Perhaps there are differences in the biology of depression in younger people; perhaps the chemical pathways that these drugs affect are less developed in the immature brain and thus less responsive to these medications. What is clear, however, is that tricyclic antidepressants must be prescribed with caution in young people and probably should not be the first choice among antidepressant medications, especially since, as you will see in the next section, safer medications with more clearly proven effectiveness are now available.

SELECTIVE SEROTONIN REUPTAKE INHIBITORS

A new pharmaceutical that had none of the tricyclics' side effects and was not toxic in overdose caused something of a sensation when it was introduced in 1988. That pharmaceutical was fluoxetine (Prozac), and "sensation" sums up the response to this medication quite well. A Prozac capsule showed up on the covers of *Newsweek* and *New York* magazines, the drug was featured in many other magazines and newspaper articles, and for a time it seemed that nearly everyone was either taking Prozac or reading the book *Listening to Prozac* (or *Talking Back to Prozac* or *Prozac Nation*). Prozac was touted by some as a miracle drug that was going to change the world.

The inevitable backlash to this enthusiasm took about another year to fully develop, but once it did, psychiatrists couldn't *pay* their patients to take Prozac. Full-page ads in *USA Today* denouncing the drug appeared for weeks, and various talk show hosts found people who gladly came on national television to swear that Prozac had made their lives miserable.

Eventually, the pendulum of public (and professional) opinion swung back towards the middle and the facts emerged. Prozac and the similar pharmaceuticals that have since been introduced are extremely safe and have a record of side effects vastly superior to that of tricyclic antidepressants. The most encouraging fact in the treatment of serious depression in young people is that, unlike the tricyclics, this group of medications has shown unequivocal benefits in double-blind placebo-controlled studies in children and adolescents.

Unlike the tricyclics, these new antidepressants have little direct effect on norepinephrine in the brain; instead, they block the reuptake of another neurotransmitter into neurons, another amine compound called *serotonin*. The very potent and specific blockade of serotonin reuptake by these agents gives this class its name: *selective serotonin reuptake inhibitors*, or *SSRIs*. As with the tricyclics, the effect on serotonin in the synapse seems to occur at the receptors, and there is some evidence that serotonin is actually the more important neurotransmitter in the treatment of depression. The development of these new agents, which help with depression but which seem to work differently from the tricyclics, has provided more clues to the underlying biology of the mood disorders.

Unlike most other psychiatric medications, most of the SSRIs have FDA-approved dosing guidelines for children and adolescents. In many cases, this approval was given several years after the drugs were labeled for use in

Table 6-2 Selective Serotonin Reuptake Inhibitors (SSRIs)

Generic Name	Brand Name
Citalopram	Celexa
Fluoxetine	Prozac
Fluvoxamine	Luvox
Paroxetine	Paxil
Sertraline	Zoloft

adults, again proving the point that off-label prescribing is not unusual for psychiatric medications in young people.

The main side effect of the SSRIs is gastrointestinal discomfort. Many patients experience nausea for the first couple of days after starting to take one of the SSRIs, and a few have diarrhea or vomiting. Fortunately, such side effects tend to pass quickly. These medications (especially fluoxetine) are also somewhat stimulating in some patients, and while this is just what some depressed people need, others feel unpleasantly nervous or "wired" on these medications. The converse can also be seen, with sleepiness sometimes a side effect. Many patients report that SSRIs seem to curb their appetite a bit, and they also notice some weight loss, especially early on in taking an SSRI. This is, of course, a potential concern in young people who are still growing. Someone who is going to have these side effects usually notices them immediately; none of them sneak up on a person who has been taking an SSRI for weeks or months.

In adults, SSRIs have been reported to cause an unpleasant blunting of emotions such that patients complain of being apathetic and indifferent to events, of being unable to get excited or enthusiastic about anything.[6] This appears to be a problem only at high doses and does not very often trouble patients taking the usual antidepressant dose.

Another side effect that has been described in adults is a change in sexual functioning, specifically a noticeable decrease in sexual interest (loss of libido) or difficulty in reaching or inability to reach orgasm. The frequency of these problems was at first difficult to gauge, because these sorts of side effects were often not asked about during clinical trials. But as more people have been treated with SSRIs since they were introduced in the early 1990s, it has become apparent that this is a significant problem affecting at least one-third of patients. I don't want to get into a discussion of the compli-

Table 6-3 More New Antidepressants

Generic Name	Brand Name
Bupropion	Wellbutrin
Mirtazapine	Remeron
Nefazodone	Serzone
Venlafaxine	Effexor

cated issue of adolescent sexuality here, but few would disagree that these are side effects that can cause significant distress. Various strategies are available for dealing with these problems when they occur, so the patient should report them to the physician. Weekend "vacations" from the medication have been reported to be helpful, as well as the addition of other medications that seem to block these effects, but sometimes a switch to another antidepressant in another class is the only solution.

Like most psychiatric medications, SSRIs are metabolized in the liver, and the details of this process have been studied more carefully for this class of medications than for most other psychiatric drugs. Many SSRIs cause a partial blockade of the cellular machinery responsible for breaking down many different medications in the liver, so they can increase the time it takes for the body to get rid of medications. This means that levels of those medications in the body will rise. For example, if an adolescent who is taking theophylline (Theo-Dur, and others) for asthma starts taking fluvoxamine (Luvox) for depression, her level of theophylline can rise to toxic levels because the antidepressant slows down theophylline metabolism. For this reason, *all* physicians caring for a patient need to know about any change of medications; they need to pay close attention to drug interactions with SSRIs—and for that matter, with all medications.

OTHER NEW ANTIDEPRESSANTS

Since the early 1990s, a whole series of new antidepressants have come on the market that are neither tricyclics nor SSRIs. Most of these pharmaceuticals don't share many common features, so there isn't a very good class name for them; you'll sometimes see many of these new agents listed as "atypical" or "second-generation" antidepressants. They have a variety of effects on norepinephrine, serotonin, and even other neurotransmitters; some have more than one effect on these systems, so they are thought to

Table 6-4 Monoamine Oxidase Inhibitors
(MAOIs)

Generic Name	Brand Name
Phenelzine	Nardil
Selegiline	Eldepryl
Tranylcypromine	Parnate

provide different ways of manipulating the chemical systems in the brain that are concerned with mood. Their side-effect profiles vary widely: some are more like tricyclics, others more like SSRIs.

Almost no data exist on the use of these medications in adolescents, and prescription of these drugs is usually off-label.

MONOAMINE OXIDASE INHIBITORS

You've already heard about iproniazid, the drug developed for the treatment of tuberculosis that caused mood elevation in some patients who took it for their lung disease. In addition to its effect on the tubercle bacillus, iproniazid causes inactivation of an enzyme in the body that metabolizes amine compounds in the nervous system. This enzyme, called *monoamine oxidase*, is responsible for gobbling up molecules of norepinephrine, serotonin, and several other neurotransmitters. Inactivating it has the effect of increasing the amounts of these compounds in the nervous system, and this effect, in some as yet poorly understood way, may be the mechanism by which these medications alleviate the symptoms of depression. This effect on the enzyme gives this class of pharmaceuticals their name: *monoamine oxidase inhibitors,* or *MAOIs.*

Monoamine oxidase is also present in the lining of the intestine and in the liver; a number of naturally occurring substances in foods are close enough chemically to norepinephrine to need deactivation before they are absorbed into the bloodstream. The importance of this becomes clear when I tell you that another name for norepinephrine is "nor*adrenaline*." Tyramine, an amino acid that has adrenaline-like effects on blood pressure and heart rate, is present in high enough concentrations in some foods to cause dangerous cardiovascular problems in persons taking MAOIs. A number of pharmaceuticals, including the ingredients of many over-the-counter reme-

Table 6-5 Foods to Avoid while Taking MAOIs

Fava or broad beans

Aged cheese (cream and cottage cheese permitted)

Beef liver or chicken liver

Orange pulp

Pickled or smoked fish, poultry, or other meats

Sauerkraut

Packaged soups

Fermented bean curd (tofu)

Yeast and protein dietary supplements

Summer (dry) sausage (e.g., pepperoni)

Soy sauce

Sour cream

Draft beer and many wines

Note: This list is not exhaustive, and some items included here are low enough in tyramine that some physicians allow one or two servings per day. Patients, and parents, should get a complete list and discuss the specifics of the diet with a knowledgeable physician, pharmacist, or nutritionist before starting to take an MAOI.

dies, also have adrenaline-like effects. Persons taking MAOIs therefore need to observe certain dietary restrictions and, even more importantly, need to *scrupulously* read the labels of any over-the-counter medication they are considering—or better yet, consult their pharmacist before taking any pharmaceutical bought over the counter.

Medications of this type also interact with other drugs that are prescribed or commonly used in emergency rooms for various problems. Anyone taking an MAOI must be sure to inform all his treating physicians that he is using this medication. He should also consider wearing an alerting bracelet so that, if he is brought unconscious to an emergency room after an accident or sudden illness, the ER personnel will be aware that he's taking an MAOI.

Other side effects accompany MAOIs too. These medications can be stimulating and cause nervousness, insomnia, and excess perspiration. Dizzy spells, especially when suddenly getting up from lying down, can occur. MAOIs block a blood pressure reflex that usually maintains blood pressure when we stand up, and the sudden drop in blood pressure on standing (called orthostatic hypotension) causes light-headedness. Weight gain, water retention, and sexual dysfunction may also occur.

As you might predict from the foregoing discussion, MAOIs are seldom used in the United States unless other antidepressants have failed to be effective, and they are even more rarely used in adolescents. Indeed, taking a medication that would mean not eating pepperoni pizzas seems too much to ask of a teenager. Nevertheless, MAOIs are sometimes uniquely effective treatments for depression. I think every psychiatrist I've ever spoken with has had the experience of effectively treating a particular patient with an MAOI after no other antidepressant had helped.

ANTIDEPRESSANT THERAPY: SOME GENERAL CONSIDERATIONS

A 1999 guide to child and adolescent psychiatry published by the American Psychiatric Association Press notes in the section on antidepressant medications that "remarkably few empirical data on children and adolescents are available to guide therapeutic choices [among the different antidepressants] and experts disagree."[7] The safety and effectiveness of the SSRIs are perhaps the most clearly supported by research, but which SSRI should be chosen as the first-line drug? What dose should be used? How long does one wait before deciding that a medication isn't working? What then?

When studies have compared antidepressant medications in large groups of (adult) patients for the treatment of depression, no single pharmaceutical has ever been proved to work better or faster that any other. There is no "best" antidepressant. If there were, we wouldn't find several dozen different ones on the market in the United States. Neither is there a "strongest" antidepressant medication. The usual dose of one may be higher, in milligrams, than that of another, but this has nothing to do with effectiveness.

I've already mentioned the evidence for superior efficacy of SSRIs over tricyclics in adolescents, but we have no evidence that one SSRI is superior to another. Considerable evidence suggests that some adult patients who get better with tricyclic medications do not improve on taking SSRIs, and vice versa. The same could well be true for adolescents: there may be a small group of adolescents for whom tricyclic medications are *more* effective than SSRIs, but the proportion of these patients to other patients responsive only to SSRIs is so small that statistical analysis doesn't "see" them in the studies done so far.

Because of this lack of proven superiority of any particular agent, subtle differences in what are, in fact, side effects are often used to make a choice among antidepressant medications. An antidepressant that is mildly sedating might be a good choice if insomnia or anxiety is a prominent symptom of depression in a particular patient. One that tends to be somewhat stimulating might be a choice if the patient is lethargic and having problems with energy level. One that stimulates appetite might be a major problem for one adolescent but just what is needed for another. The physician's experience with a particular medication may make it a "first among equals" in her prescribing for patients. Indeed, a medication that a particular doctor has had a lot of experience with in prescribing for patients probably *is* a better medicine than a very similar one that she hasn't prescribed very much—for this doctor's patients at least.

I've already discussed some of the problems in deciding on a dose for adolescents. Fortunately, more data are becoming available all the time to help with this. Most of the SSRIs are already labeled for use in young patients. Remember, too, that depression in older adolescents is usually not so different from that seen in adults, and probably little alteration in treatment will be needed from that used for adults. No radical biological shift occurs on an adolescent's eighteenth birthday that makes him suddenly an adult physiologically. Treatment decisions for some 17- and 16-year-olds may be the same as those for adults.

One of the most frustrating aspects of antidepressant therapy is the lag time between starting medication and improvement in symptoms. Most studies of depressed patients first starting to take an antidepressant medication report some improvement of symptoms within two weeks. But it often takes longer for improvement to be noticed. The sequence of events brought about in the brain by antidepressant treatment most likely involves a re-engineering of neurons on some level, probably through the turning on of genes in these cells. This process takes time. It's not unreasonable to wait for four to six weeks before giving up on a medication. Even when a medication is beginning to help, it may take a long time for its *full* benefit to become apparent. Studies of depressed adults indicate that depressive symptoms continue to improve for up to three months after starting to take antidepressant medications.

What options are available if a medication doesn't seem to be helping? Raising the dose is often the first choice. A switch to an antidepressant in a different class is another. At some point, adding another medication is often tried. Some patients respond to combinations of antidepressants or a combination of an antidepressant and another type of medication, such as a mood-stabilizing medication.

We have no way to know beforehand which patient will respond to which antidepressant. And we have no way to know which, if any, side effects a particular person will develop. Unfortunately, some trial and error is required in the process of finding the medication or combination of medications that works best with the least side effects. The prescribing of antidepressant medications can accurately be described as an art rather than a science, at least for now.

CHAPTER 7

Mood-Stabilizing Medications

M ood stabilizers are medications that have both antimanic and antidepressant effects. They are usually the foundation for the treatment of people with bipolar disorders, and they are used for other
problems as well. Mood stabilizers, especially lithium, are often used in
combination with antidepressant medications to treat depression that is unresponsive to an antidepressant alone. At the end of this chapter, I'll discuss
how physicians go about making the decision to treat an individual with a
mood stabilizer.

LITHIUM

In the second century A.D., the Greek physician Soranus of Ephesus recommended that physicians treating patients suffering from mania should
prescribe "natural waters, such as [from] alkaline springs."[1] Roman physicians recommended that their patients "take the waters" at various springs
for a whole variety of physical and mental ailments. The little town of Spa
in eastern Belgium, Bath in England, Wiesbaden in Germany, and dozens
of other towns in Italy and Greece that were the sites of natural springs became centers for healing. As the science of analytical chemistry developed,
curious chemists and physicians evaluated these various springs and found
that the waters of many were rich in lithium.

In the middle of the nineteenth century, lithium compounds were tried
as treatments for gout and kidney stones. Unfortunately, the approach was

unsuccessful and was soon abandoned. Nevertheless, this work led to formulation of pharmaceutical preparations of lithium compounds and to information on the range of safe doses for lithium preparations in humans.

In the 1940s, lithium came to medical attention again when lithium chloride was introduced as a substitute for table salt (sodium chloride) for people with medical problems, such as heart disease and high blood pressure, that required them to be on a low-sodium diet. But when heart patients were given saltshakers full of lithium salts to sprinkle on their food, the results were catastrophic for some. Because lithium is toxic in surprisingly low concentrations, substituting lithium chloride for sodium chloride turned out to be a disaster. There were many reports of severe lithium poisoning and even several deaths. The use of lithium as a salt substitute ended, and the episode had the effect of giving lithium a very bad reputation among physicians.

So it was very much a chance occurrence that led to the discovery of lithium's beneficial effects on mood disorders in 1948. John F. J. Cade, M.D., senior medical officer in the Mental Hygiene Department of Victoria, Australia, was working in his laboratory on trying to determine whether some toxin might be present in the urine of individuals with manic-depressive illness. Cade was especially interested in urea and uric acid, by-products of protein metabolism found in urine, and was testing the toxicity of these compounds by injecting small amounts of them into guinea pigs.

One of the technical problems with his work was that uric acid is rather insoluble in water, making it difficult to prepare injectable solutions of higher concentrations. Looking for a soluble urate salt to use instead of uric acid, Cade consulted prior research and discovered that uric acid was easiest to dissolve in water when it was combined with lithium as lithium urate. He injected small amounts of lithium urate into the guinea pigs and noticed that uric acid seemed to be much less toxic in this form. This suggested to Cade that the lithium component of the compound might have some sort of protective effect against urate toxicity. To determine what the effect of the lithium ion might be, he injected lithium carbonate (the carbonate ion is a harmless substance, found, for example, as sodium carbonate in baking soda)[2] and discovered that "after a latent period of about two hours the animals, although fully conscious, became extremely lethargic and unresponsive to stimuli for one to two hours before once again becoming normally active."[3]

As Cade admitted in his original paper, "It may seem a long distance from lethargy in guinea pigs to excitement in psychotics,"[4] but doctors of the time were desperate for new treatment possibilities. So Cade decided to administer lithium preparations to several patients who were chronically agitated. The effect on individuals with mania was dramatic:

CASE I—W.B., a male aged fifty-one years, who had been in a state of chronic manic excitement for five years, restless, dirty, destructive, mischievous and interfering, had long been regarded as the most troublesome patient in the ward. His response was highly gratifying. From the start of treatment on March 29, 1948, with lithium citrate he steadily settled down and in three weeks was enjoying the unaccustomed surrounding of the convalescent ward. As he had been ill so long and confined to a "chronic ward," he found normal surroundings and liberty of movement strange at first. He remained perfectly well and left the hospital on indefinite leave with instructions to take a dose of lithium carbonate, five grains, twice a day. He was soon back working at his old job.

CASE VIII—W.M., a man of fifty years, was suffering from an attack of recurrent mania, the first of which he had had at the age of twenty. The present attack had lasted two months and showed no signs of abating. He was garrulous, euphoric, restless and unkempt when he started taking lithium. Two days later he was reported to be quieter. By the ninth day he was definitely settling down and the following day commenced work in the garden. By the end of two weeks he was practically normal—quiet, tidy, rational, with insight into his previous condition.[5]

At this point, Dr. Cade had treated ten manic patients with lithium, and all ten had shown the same dramatic improvement. One would think the news of Cade's discovery would have spread like wildfire. It did not. In fact, not until several decades later did the United States Food and Drug Administration approve lithium for the treatment of bipolar disorder. Part of the reason for this delay was the state of world psychiatry following the end of the Second World War. Much of European psychiatry, especially German psychiatry, was in ruins, literally and figuratively. In the United States and England, psychoanalytic theories had replaced the traditional medical practices of evaluation, diagnosis, and treatment with the prescription of "the talking cure" for all emotional problems. Accurate psychiatric diagnosis simply didn't exist. Ronald Fieve, the American psychiatrist who would champion the use of lithium in the United States in the 1970s and who was instrumental in getting American psychiatrists to prescribe it for their patients, observed that, during the late 1940s and the 1950s in New York, he "rarely met with the diagnosis of manic-depression . . . It had virtually disappeared. Most cases of excitable, talkative, and elated behavior were being diagnosed as schizophrenia."[6]

But a Danish psychiatrist, Morgans Schou, realized that Cade's discovery represented a real breakthrough (noting in a 1954 paper that "it is rather astonishing that [Cade's] observation has failed to arouse greater general interest among psychiatrists").[7] Schou very quickly became convinced of the effectiveness of lithium in treating acute mania, and he was one of the first clinical researchers to become convinced of another therapeutic effect of the drug: its ability to prevent further episodes of illness (lithium's preventive, or *prophylactic*, effect). Schou had a more difficult time convincing his colleagues around the world that lithium could prevent recurrences of bipolar disorder and that patients should take it even after their acute symptoms had subsided. In 1967, Schou and his colleague Paul Christian Baalstrup reported on eighty-eight patients who had taken lithium for several years and had experienced a dramatic reduction in the frequency and duration of their mood episodes. Several patients who had been sick for several weeks out of every year experienced a complete remission of their illness that lasted for more than five years: their illness had essentially stopped.[8]

As Schou and his colleagues treated more and more patients with lithium, their findings that lithium favorably altered the course of bipolar illness became so clear that they had ethical qualms about doing a more rigorous placebo-controlled study—one in which patients with bipolar disorder would be divided into two groups, some to receive lithium and the others a placebo. Several British psychiatrists scolded the Danes for reporting their results without a placebo-controlled study, so Baalstrup and Schou did a lithium discontinuation study in which they selected patients who had been stable while taking lithium for at least a year, divided them into two roughly equal groups, and in one group substituted a placebo for the lithium. The results were dramatic: of the thirty-nine participants whose lithium was replaced with the placebo, twenty-one relapsed within five months; *none* of the forty-five participants still taking lithium had a relapse.

It took a few more years to show that lithium is an effective antidepressant as well, but by the early 1980s, clinical studies had clearly shown that

	Depression
|||||||	Mania
——	Lithium administration

Figure 7-1 This graph illustrates data from six patients in Baalstrup and Schou's early study of the protective effect of lithium against the relapse of bipolar symptoms. Each line represents the symptom course of one patient. In all these patients, when lithium was started, episodes of depression and mania stopped completely.

Source: Data from Paul Baalstrup and Morgans Schou, "Lithium as a Prophylactic Agent: Its Effect against Recurrent Depressions and Manic-Depressive Psychosis," *Archives of General Psychiatry* 16, no. 2 (1967): 162–72.

lithium is also effective in the treatment of depressive syndrome.[9] Also clearly proven is that adding lithium to antidepressant medication can benefit people who have had an incomplete response to an antidepressant. This use, often referred to as antidepressant *augmentation,* can effectively turn a poor or incomplete therapeutic effect into a complete one.[10]

Therapeutic Profile

Lithium is a naturally occurring element found in mineral springs, seawater, and certain ores. Like its close cousin, sodium, it is never found in its pure form in nature, but rather combined with other ions as a salt of one type or another. It is mined on an industrial scale for use in the manufacture of ceramics and batteries. Therapeutic lithium preparations usually contain lithium carbonate.

Because it is an element, lithium is not metabolized within the body,

Table 7-1 Therapeutic Profile of Lithium

Medication class:	Mood stabilizer
Brand names:	Eskalith, Eskalith CR, Lithobid, Lithonate, Lithotabs
Generic names:	Lithium carbonate, lithium citrate (liquid preparation)
Half-life:	14–30 hours
Metabolism:	None
Need for birth control:	Probably mandatory (see text)
Other considerations:	Blood levels extremely important

and because lithium ions are so similar to sodium ions, the body handles lithium in much the same way it handles sodium. Lithium is rapidly absorbed through the gastrointestinal tract, enters the bloodstream, and is eliminated from the body by being filtered out by the kidneys.

Descriptions of the effects of a pharmaceutical in the body always include a vital statistic called its *half-life*. This is a measure of how quickly the body gets rid of a medication. Specifically, it is the time required for half the amount of the drug to be eliminated or metabolized by the body. Put another way, it is the time the body takes to reduce the level of the medication by half. The half-life of lithium in children and adolescents is about the same as in adults: approximately eighteen hours.[11] Another useful number, which can be derived from the half-life statistic for any medication, is the time required for the level of medication to build up to a constant level in the body—the time required for the amount taken in to equal the amount eliminated: the equilibrium point. By a series of mathematical steps that we don't need to detail here, it can be shown that the equilibrium point is the same for all medications: five half-lives. This means that, since the half-life of lithium is roughly one day, it takes roughly five days for lithium, when first taken, to reach a steady level in the bloodstream. It also means that if the lithium dose is changed, it takes about five days for the blood level to stabilize at a new level.

Because of the toxic effects and even deaths that were reported when heart patients sprinkled lithium salt freely on their food, there was a significant delay in the acceptance of lithium as a therapeutic agent. Lithium is a powerful pharmaceutical, one that must be treated with respect. It has a very low *therapeutic index*, meaning that the difference between the ther-

Table 7-2 Comparison of Higher and Lower Lithium Levels in Relapse Rates of Bipolar Disorder

Treatment Group	Any Relapse	Depressed	Mixed/ Manic	Hypomanic	Withdrew from Study
Standard dose range (0.8–1.0 meq/L)	6 (12%)	3 (6%)	3 (6%)	0	24 (51%)
Low dose range (0.4–0.6 meq/L)	21 (44%)	1 (2%)	17 (35%)	3 (6%)	11 (23%)

Source: Data from Alan Gelenberg, John Kane, Martin Keller, Phillip Lavori, Jerrold Rosenbaum, Karyl Cole, and Janet Lavelle, "Comparison of Standard and Low Levels of Lithium for Maintenance Treatment of Bipolar Disorder," *New England Journal of Medicine* 321, no. 22 (1989): 1489–93.

apeutic dose and a toxic dose is small.[12] Fortunately, lithium can be measured in the bloodstream accurately and fairly cheaply, and the dosage adjusted accordingly.

Monitoring of lithium levels in the blood is important not only to prevent toxicity but also because clinical studies have clearly demonstrated that, for most individuals, lithium needs to be present in the bloodstream at a certain level to be effective.[13] Clinical studies indicate that the therapeutic range for maximum efficacy is the same in adolescents and adults. But just what that level should be has been a matter of some debate.

An important study from the Massachusetts General Hospital found that a level of between 0.8 and 1.0 meq/L (milliequivalent per liter, a chemical measure of concentration) was most effective. In this double-blind study, adults with bipolar disorder were divided into two groups: a "standard dose" group, whose lithium levels were kept between 0.8 and 1.0 meq/L, and a "low dose" group, whose levels were maintained between 0.4 and 0.6 meq/L. The result was that the relapse rate in the "low dose" group was more than double that in the "standard dose" group (see table 7-2).

There is more to these data than may initially meet the eye, however. Many more patients from the "standard dose" group than from the "low dose" group dropped out of the study because of side effects. The take-home message seems to be that levels closer to 1.0 meq/L are more protective—but that many people have trouble taking such a high dose because of side effects. Many psychiatrists compromise and try to maintain their patients at levels between these two. Dr. Schou, whom many consider the father of lithium therapy, has recommended levels of 0.5 to 0.8 meq/L for the treatment of bipolar disorder in adults.[14] However, it's very clear that some people have good control of their symptoms with even lower levels, elderly persons for example. Lithium levels thus need to be individualized for individual patients, and as Dr. Schou also points out, "Changes in lithium levels as small as 0.1 to 0.2 [meq/L], upward or downward, may substantially improve patients' quality of life during maintenance treatment."[15]

The lithium level rises in the bloodstream after every dose, peaks in about two hours, and then begins to fall again. If a patient takes his lithium two or three times a day, there will be several peaks and valleys. Because the level is rising and falling throughout the day, in checking lithium level it is important that the blood be drawn at a time when the result can be correctly interpreted. The convention that has been adopted is to use a twelve-hour level, making it convenient to draw blood in the mornings. For most patients this means getting to the lab twelve hours after their bedtime dose (for example, at 11 A.M., if the bedtime dose was at 11 P.M. the night before), without having taken their usual morning dose.

Lithium is approved for use in the treatment of bipolar disorder in adolescents over the age of 12. Given what I've said about the variability of physical maturity in adolescents, you may wonder why the FDA doesn't label lithium and other drugs as approved for people of a certain height or weight rather than a certain age. The short answer is that this is simply how the FDA decided to do things. Remember that pharmaceutical labeling is a *guide* to prescribing medications, not "rules" for prescribing them.

Clinical research indicates that lithium is as effective for the treatment of bipolar disorder in adolescents as it is in adults.[16] The research on using lithium as an augmentation of antidepressant treatment is more limited for adolescents than for adults, but the results are very encouraging. In open trials of lithium as an augmentation of tricyclic antidepressants, about half the adolescents who had not had an adequate response to a tricyclic alone got better when lithium was added. This is about the same response usually seen in adults.[17] There have been case reports of lithium also helping the newer antidepressants to work better.[18]

Side Effects

Individuals vary widely in their sensitivity to side effects of lithium (and of all medications, for that matter). Some people have none; others have sev-

Table 7-3 Treatable Side Effects of Lithium

Side Effect	Remedy
Nausea, diarrhea	Take immediately after meals; switch to a controlled-release preparation
Weight gain	Diet and exercise
Tremor	Cut out caffeine-containing beverages; take beta-blocker medications
Flare-up of preexisting dermatological condition	Dermatological preparations
Hypothyroidism	Thyroid medications

eral. Fortunately, almost all of lithium's side effects can be eliminated or managed.

Many of the side effects are *dose-related*: the higher the lithium dose, the more severe the side effect. One management strategy, then, is simply to lower the lithium dose. The advantages of higher levels are clear, as noted above, but most physicians will aim to maintain patients at the lowest possible dose that controls their symptoms.

Because of its similarity to sodium, lithium has some of the same effects that an increased sodium (table salt) intake would have: increased thirst, increased urination, and water retention. These side effects are often temporary and subside as the body adjusts to the medication. If they do not, the judicious use of medications that promote urination and excretion of excess body water (diuretics) can help. DO NOT ALLOW YOUR CHILD TO TAKE DIURETICS WITHOUT CONSULTING A PHYSICIAN! Some diuretics have the effect of raising lithium levels and can cause severe lithium toxicity. The regular lithium dose must usually be lowered and blood levels of lithium must be scrupulously monitored if a patient takes diuretics regularly. There have been reports of persistent and severe increased urination ("diabetes insipidus," which has nothing to do with "diabetes mellitus," the common "sugar diabetes") that progresses over time. Also, a few cases of impaired kidney functioning have been reported. Both these problems are rare and slow to develop. Nevertheless, in addition to monitoring lithium levels, blood tests that measure kidney functioning are routinely ordered for patients taking lithium.

Lithium is irritating to the gastrointestinal tract and can cause nausea or diarrhea; taking it on a full stomach can ease these problems considerably. A fine shaking in the hands (tremor) can occur at higher lithium levels; medications used to treat tremors, called beta-blockers, are frequently prescribed and can be very helpful. Weight gain can be a very annoying side effect and unfortunately has an equally annoying remedy: diet and exercise.

Between 5 and 35 percent of people treated with lithium develop depression of thyroid gland functioning (hypothyroidism).[19] A test of thyroid functioning is the third in the battery of blood tests routinely ordered for persons taking lithium.

Lithium can cause flare-ups of preexisting skin conditions, but only rarely causes the new onset of dermatological problems. Individuals with acne, psoriasis, or other dermatological problems may need closer follow-up from their dermatologist.

Because those who start taking lithium for a mood disorder as an adolescent will often continue doing so into adulthood, it's important to note that lithium has been associated with birth defects. Remember that by the time a woman misses her period after conceiving, development of many of the embryo's major organs is already well under way. Stopping a medication after a woman *knows* she is pregnant may well be too late to prevent a birth defect. Women of childbearing age have usually been advised to practice birth control while taking lithium, if there is any chance of becoming pregnant. Some more recent data suggest that children born to women taking lithium have only a slightly increased chance of birth defects. Women taking lithium who want to get pregnant should have a discussion with their psychiatrist and obstetrician about the risks of taking lithium and of stopping lithium. There is still disagreement about which course is riskier. Lithium is secreted in breast milk, and women taking lithium should not breast-feed.

Another of lithium's side effects that troubles a significant number of people is a noticeable dulling of mental functioning. Patients complain that their ability to memorize and learn is affected and that they have a difficult-to-describe sense of mental sluggishness. For years, clinicians downplayed these complaints as coming from people who simply weren't used to being "normal," individuals who just missed the mental hyper-alertness of hypomania. This view seemed to be supported by research using psychological tests on persons taking lithium for the treatment of bipolar disorder, research that has been basically inconclusive. But when nonpatient volunteers were administered lithium and similarly tested, a small but definite drop off in their performance was found,[20] proving that this lithium-induced mental sluggishness is a very real problem for some people. This side effect should be checked into for adolescents who seem to be having difficulties in school, even though their mood problem is under better control. This is a dose-related side effect and is another reason to strive for the lowest possible maintenance dose of lithium that still controls mood symptoms adequately.

VALPROATE (DEPAKOTE)

The development of valproate (brand names include Depakote and Depakene) for the treatment of mood disorders is another convoluted study in serendipity. Valproic acid is a carbon-containing compound similar to a number of others that are found in animal fats and vegetable oils: a fatty acid. It was first synthesized in 1882 and used as an organic solvent (a liquid in which other substances dissolve) for many years, for a variety of purposes. Many decades ago, pharmacists used it as a solvent for bismuth salts, which were used to treat stomach and skin disorders.

In the early 1960s, scientists looking for treatments for epilepsy were working with a group of new pharmaceutical compounds that appeared promising but were difficult to dissolve. They discovered that valproic acid was an effective solvent for the compounds they were testing, and they started using it to dissolve their test drugs for animal experimentation. As they tested their various new pharmaceuticals, the results they obtained seemed confusing—until someone realized that it didn't matter *which* of the new pharmaceuticals was used. As long as *any* of them was dissolved in valproic acid, the drug was found to be effective in stopping epileptic seizure activity. It soon became obvious that the valproic acid was stopping the seizures, not what was dissolved in it. By 1978, valproate was approved by the FDA for use in treating epilepsy.[21]

In the 1960s, there were some reports that valproate might be helpful in mood disorders, and throughout the late 1960s and early 1970s a French psychiatrist named Lambert published a series of papers about using it to treat bipolar disorders. After the discovery that another antiepilepsy medication, carbamazepine, was effective in treating mania, interest in the possibilities of valproate as a mood stabilizer grew. In the mid-1980s, several studies on the use of valproate in treating bipolar disorder were published by American psychiatrists, and ten years later, valproate had become firmly established as an effective antimanic medication and a mood stabilizer in adults; it is now FDA-approved for use in bipolar disorder (in adults). Less research has been done on adolescents, but the available data indicate that valproate is effective for adolescents with bipolar disorder. Because one of valproate's first uses was for seizure disorders in children and adolescents, there is a large amount of information on dosing, safety, and side effects in young people.

Valproate's therapeutic action in bipolar disorder (or in epilepsy, for that matter) is still completely unknown. We do know that it improves neuronal transmission in the brain that is mediated by the neurotransmitter *gamma-aminobutyric acid* (GABA). GABA seems to have an inhibitory or modulating effect on many brain circuits, and valproate's effect may be to enhance this modulator in some way.

Therapeutic Profile

Valproate is known to be effective in the treatment of acute mania. It also appears to be effective in preventing the recurrence, and reducing the severity, of episodes of bipolar disorder. Its effectiveness in the treatment of acute depressive episodes of bipolar disorder has been less impressive.

In reading about this medication, you'll notice the many names it goes by: valproate, valproic acid, divalproex sodium, not to mention the brand names, Depakote and Depakene. Valproate is the name of the negative ion. When associated with a hydrogen ion, the result is valproic acid; in combination with a sodium ion it becomes sodium valproate. Depakote, a preparation manufactured by Abbott Laboratories, consists of a stable combination of sodium valproate and valproic acid called divalproex sodium. (Depakene is Abbott's brand name for their valproic acid preparation.)

Valproate seems to be more effective than lithium for certain subgroups of patients: those with rapid cycling (four or more mood episodes per year) and those with mixed mania, that is, a mixture of manic hyperactivity and pressured thinking and depressed or unpleasant mood.[22] Also, valproate is much less toxic than lithium. One big disadvantage of valproate is that it does not seem to be as helpful as lithium in treating acute depression. Nor is it very effective in preventing recurrences of depression.[23] This suggests that valproate may be a better choice for individuals with rapid cycling or with mixed mania, but that those with classic euphoric mania and major depression may have better control of their symptoms with lithium.[24]

Table 7-4	Therapeutic Profile of Valproate
Medication class:	Mood stabilizer (anticonvulsant)
Brand names:	Depakote, Depakene
Generic names:	Divalproex sodium, valproic acid
Half-life:	6–16 hours
Metabolism:	Affected by other antiepilepsy drugs
Elimination:	By liver and kidneys
Need for birth control:	Probably mandatory
Other considerations:	Blood levels helpful to adjust dose; blood tests for liver inflammation needed

Like lithium, valproate can be measured in the bloodstream; unfortunately, it is more difficult to measure and requires a more expensive test. Blood levels above 45 mcg/mL (micrograms per milliliter) have been shown to be necessary for the therapeutic effect to occur, and side effects become more problematic at levels greater than 125 mcg/mL.[25] Several studies have shown that valproate is helpful in cyclothymia, bipolar II, and "soft" bipolar disorders and that lower doses and lower blood levels are required than in the treatment of bipolar I.[26] As with lithium, in measuring valproate levels, blood should be drawn twelve hours after the last dose of medication.

Valproate has also been used to treat more general behavioral problems in children and adolescents, specifically impulse problems, aggressiveness, and severe temper tantrums.[27] Valproate has significant antianxiety effects and is sometimes prescribed for this reason, especially in Europe.

Side Effects

Valproate has a milder side-effect profile than lithium and is not nearly as toxic in overdose. Side effects that are common as an individual starts taking the medication include stomach upset and some sleepiness. These problems usually go away quickly. Increased appetite and weight gain can occur. Mild tremor also occurs and can be treated with beta-blocker medication. A few patients report hair loss, usually temporary, which resolves even more quickly with vitamin preparations containing the minerals zinc and selenium.[28] Most dandruff shampoos contain selenium, and these help combat this type of hair loss too.

Cases of severe liver problems have been reported in patients taking valproate. These occurred almost exclusively in young children (under age 2) taking the drug for control of epilepsy, most of whom had other medical problems and were taking several different medications. A 1989 review article stated that no fatalities from liver problems caused by valproate had ever been reported for individuals over the age of 10 who were taking only valproate.[29] Just to be on the safe side, however, a blood test that can detect liver inflammation is done for those taking valproate for the first time and is repeated at appropriate intervals while they are taking this medication. Because valproate also, though rarely, causes a drop in blood cell count, a complete blood count is usually done as well. These are very rare problems. Even when they do occur, they develop slowly and usually during the first six months of therapy, and thus can be picked up with routine blood tests. Nevertheless, individuals taking valproate should be on the lookout for signs of liver or blood count problems: unusual bleeding and bruising, jaundice (yellowing of the eyes and skin), fever, and water retention.

Valproate has been associated with birth defects and, as with lithium, women in the childbearing years should practice birth control while taking valproate if there is any possibility of becoming pregnant. There is also controversy about the frequency with which valproate causes multiple ovarian cysts (polycystic ovaries) in women who have taken it for many years. One expert's review of the situation estimated that up to 80 percent of female patients who started taking valproate before the age of 20 had some kind of hormonal problems.[30] This is an important consideration in prescribing this medication to adolescent girls.

CARBAMAZEPINE (TEGRETOL)

After the introduction of carbamazepine (brand names include Tegretol and Epitol) for the control of epilepsy in the 1960s, several reports appeared indicating that, when taking this medication, people with epilepsy who also had mood problems not only had good control of their seizures but had improvement in their psychiatric symptoms as well. It was a small step to test carbamazepine in patients with mood problems who did not suffer from epilepsy. Much of the earlier work on the use of carbamazepine in treating bipolar disorder was done by Japanese clinicians looking for an alternative to lithium, which was not approved for use in Japan until years after it was available in the United States. In 1980, a study appeared in the *American*

Journal of Psychiatry titled "Carbamazepine in Manic-Depressive Illness: A New Treatment."[31] Although carbamazepine has been used to treat epilepsy in children and adolescents for many years, it is currently not labeled by the FDA for the treatment of psychiatric disorders in children or adolescents (or adults, for that matter).

Therapeutic Profile

Carbamazepine is one of those medications that don't seem to have any particular advantage in most studies on groups of psychiatric patients, but it works very well—in fact, works when other medications do not—in some individuals. In one well-designed double-blind study, manic patients who took carbamazepine actually seemed to do worse than those taking lithium.[32] But most psychiatrists have had a patient like "Ms. B.," whose case history was reported in a paper from the National Institute of Mental Health in 1983:

> CASE 2. MS. B., a 53-year-old woman, had a history of treatment resistant, rapid cycling manic-depressive illness that required continuous state hospitalization from 1956 to her admission to NIMH in 1978. She had been non-responsive to [antipsychotic medications, tricyclic antidepressants] and lithium . . . After institution of carbamazepine, both mood phases improved dramatically and she was able to be discharged . . . During a subsequent hospitalization her severe mania again did not respond to [antipsychotic medications] and she was not able to leave the hospital until she was treated with carbamazepine.[33]

The authors of this study noted, "Additional improvement appeared to occur when [antipsychotic medications] were used in conjunction with carbamazepine or when lithium and carbamazepine were used in combination." This has become carbamazepine's niche: a second-line mood-stabilizing agent for patients who do not respond to other agents, often used in combination with other agents.

A series of case reports published in 1999 supports carbamazepine's effectiveness in the treatment of bipolar disorder in adolescents. The cases included a 17-year-old girl and a 14-year-old boy who had classic bipolar symptoms with severe depressions and manias. Both had only a partial response to lithium and significant side effects with it. Because of these problems, these children had stopped taking the medication several times and

Table 7-5 Therapeutic Profile of Carbamazepine

Medication class:	Mood stabilizer (anticonvulsant)
Brand names:	Epitol, Tegretol
Generic name:	Carbamazepine
Half-life:	18–55 hours (shortens after time)
Metabolism:	Complex: affects and is affected by other drugs
Elimination:	By liver and kidneys
Need for birth control:	Probably mandatory
Other considerations:	Blood levels helpful to adjust dose; blood tests for liver inflammation and blood abnormalities needed

had suffered relapses. Both had excellent remissions of their symptoms on taking carbamazepine, and because they didn't have side-effect problems they were willing to take it continuously and therefore stayed well.[34]

Like the other mood-stabilizing medications, carbamazepine can be measured in the bloodstream and the blood levels used to adjust the dose. Unfortunately, not much work has been done on blood levels of this medication in patients with bipolar disorder, so the therapeutic range used for the treatment of epilepsy is usually the target that psychiatrists aim for in their patients.

Carbamazepine is metabolized in the liver, and, like some other drugs, it causes the levels of liver enzymes that metabolize it to increase. This means that the longer a person takes carbamazepine, the better the liver becomes at getting rid of it. So after a few weeks, the blood levels of the drug may go down and the dose may need to be increased. This increase in liver enzymes can also affect other medications that the patient might be taking, including certain tranquilizers, certain antidepressants, other epilepsy medications, and some hormones, including birth-control preparations. It is very important to inform all physicians involved in a person's care that she has started taking carbamazepine, so that dosage adjustments can be made.

Side Effects

Carbamazepine can produce the sort of general side effects caused by many medications affecting the brain: sleepiness, light-headedness, and some initial nausea. These problems tend to be short-lived and dose-related.

As with valproate, there have been rare cases of liver problems, so blood tests for liver inflammation are routinely done. There have also been rare reports of dangerous changes in blood cell counts, so blood counts are also done, especially in the first several weeks of therapy. Some cases of a rare but dangerous skin reaction called Stevens-Johnson syndrome have occurred. Although all these problems are very uncommon, patients should be on the watch for the development of a rash, jaundice, water retention, bleeding or bruising, or signs of infection.

LAMOTRIGINE (LAMICTAL)

Lamotrigine (brand name Lamictal) is another antiseizure medication that appears to have therapeutic effects for people with mood disorders. Studies began to appear in the 1980s showing that it was a useful "add-on" therapy for people with epilepsy who were already taking other antiseizure medications. During the early investigations of this use, researchers noted that patients who took lamotrigine for seizure control reported an improvement in their mood and sense of well-being—even if it hadn't helped much with their seizures. Lamotrigine has several effects on the brain that might explain its efficacy in bipolar disorder. It appears to inhibit release of the neurotransmitter *glutamate*, an amino acid that causes stimulation of various neural circuits. Lamotrigine is also thought to affect at least one of the same second-messenger systems that lithium affects, the *inositol triphosphate system*.[35]

Therapeutic Profile

Because it is such a new agent, lamotrigine's place in the treatment of bipolar disorder is still unclear. The most exciting aspect of its profile is its apparent effectiveness in depression, including both bipolar and unipolar depression. One of the first reports on its use in the treatment of bipolar disorder described a patient who had suffered from rapid-cycling bipolar I disorder since he was 14.[36] In the year before starting to take lamotrigine, he had been either depressed or manic continuously with no period of normal mood. When the research team first saw him, he was severely depressed and had not responded to lithium or carbamazepine or an antidepressant. On taking lamotrigine, his depression symptoms gradually improved and, as of eleven months later, he hadn't had a recurrence of either depressive or manic symptoms. There are other reports of lamotrig-

Table 7-6 Therapeutic Profile of Lamotrigine

Medication class:	Mood stabilizer (anticonvulsant)
Brand name:	Lamictal
Generic name:	Lamotrigine
Half-life:	15–24 hours
Metabolism:	Complex: affected by other drugs
Elimination:	By liver and kidneys
Need for birth control:	Recommended
Other considerations:	Rarely causes severe skin rashes, but has a generally good side-effect profile

ine being very helpful in cases of extremely treatment-resistant major depressive disorder in adults.[37]

Other studies indicate that lamotrigine works well with other mood stabilizers in treatment-resistant patients and can sometimes turn a partial medication response into a more complete one.[38] Lamotrigine is a welcome addition to the present array of mood stabilizers—especially in the light of its apparent antidepressant effects.

Lamotrigine has a half-life of about twenty-four hours, and the body's ability to metabolize it is affected by taking carbamazepine and valproate. Blood levels are not routinely ordered for lamotrigine because of its low toxicity and because therapeutic effects have not been correlated with a particular blood-level range.

Side Effects

Aside from some initial nausea or gastrointestinal upset and the sort of side effects that many medications affecting the brain can cause—sleepiness, light-headedness or dizziness, and headache—lamotrigine has a very good side-effect profile. The most serious side effects reported are serious types of skin rashes, Stevens-Johnson syndrome and toxic epidermal necrosis (TED). This last is a very severe rash that has the effect of a whole-body third-degree burn and has been fatal in some cases. The likelihood of this problem developing has been greatly reduced by the practice of starting the medication at a very low dose and raising the dose quite gradually. Although this means it takes a lot longer (several weeks) to get to a therapeutic dose, the technique has greatly reduced the number of serious rashes. Also, the rash problem seems to be more frequently seen in individuals who have had other dermatological reactions to medications. Unfortunately, TED has been reported more often in young people than in adults, so lamotrigine is not recommended by the manufacturer for children under the age of 16. Patients should examine their skin carefully, especially during the first several weeks of therapy, and stop the medication and get in touch with their doctor at any sign of skin rash. In older adolescents with treatment-resistant depression, lamotrigine may be an option.

OTHER MOOD STABILIZERS

A number of other agents show promise for the treatment of bipolar disorder. For the most part, the promise of these medications is based on a few case reports of a therapeutic effect in adults; in some cases, they are medications in the same class as other pharmaceuticals already shown to be helpful.

Gabapentin (brand name Neurontin) is yet another antiseizure medication that seems to be a mood stabilizer as well. As with the others, reports of beneficial effects on mood disorder symptoms in people being treated for epilepsy came first, and a few indicators of effect in bipolar disorder followed. One case report concerned a man with bipolar disorder who refused to take lithium and who had liver disease and low blood counts caused by alcoholism.[39] Because he wouldn't take lithium and his medical problems made the use of valproate or carbamazepine risky, gabapentin was tried. He had a "dramatic" decrease in manic symptoms, his sleep pattern returned to normal, and best of all he reported no side effects. In another preliminary study, gabapentin was given to twenty-eight patients with various forms of bipolar disorder who had not had a satisfactory response to lithium, valproate, or carbamazepine.[40] Eighteen of the twenty-eight had a positive response. Gabapentin is not metabolized in the liver and so does not affect the blood levels of other medications; it doesn't need blood-level monitoring and has a very good side-effect profile. It remains to be seen whether gabapentin will live up to these encouraging early reports.

Oxcarbazepine (brand name Trileptal) is an antiepilepsy drug very similar to carbamazepine. Several encouraging studies from Germany were published in the 1980s describing its use in treating bipolar disorder in adults, but the drug was not approved for use in the United States until January 2000. The case of a 6-year-old girl with severe bipolar disorder who was successfully treated with oxcarbazepine appeared in the *Journal of the American Academy of Child and Adolescent Psychiatry* in 2001. This little girl had mood symptoms with severe aggression and violent behaviors that included breaking windows and knocking doors off their hinges. She had not benefited from lithium but had "full mood stabilization" after six weeks of taking oxcarbazepine. After three months, her mother reported that she was "fabulous" and her teacher said she was a "little angel."[41] Oxcarbazepine has fewer side effects than carbamazepine and has not been associated with the dangerous skin rashes and blood count problems occurring with that drug.

Other antiepilepsy drugs that have attracted the interest of clinical researchers on bipolar disorder are *topiramate* (brand name Topamax) and *tiagabine* (Gabatril). Ongoing research may result in these drugs also being introduced as mood-stabilizing medications.

WHAT DO MOOD STABILIZERS TREAT?

Research clearly indicates that lithium, valproate, carbamazepine, and probably lamotrigine are very effective for the treatment of bipolar disorder in adults, especially for mania. There are more limited studies on younger patients, but the results have been encouraging. Adding mood-stabilizing medications, primarily lithium, to an antidepressant medication for adult patients who have treatment-resistant depression is also clearly helpful and can turn a partial remission of symptoms into a complete one. Again, there is less research on this use in adolescents, but what is available supports the view that this is an effective strategy. Thus, mood-stabilizing medications seem to have a place in the management of both bipolar disorders and depressive disorders.

These medications have also been used to treat behavioral problems that have some overlap with the symptoms of mood disorders. *Conduct disorder* is a diagnosis given to children and adolescents who are aggressive, destructive, and disobedient and who break the rules and often the law with behaviors such as stealing. Many of these adolescents show symptoms of depressed or irritable mood, impulsivity, and temper tantrums and have substance-abuse problems. Several studies have looked at the effectiveness of mood-stabilizing medications for these problems; some of the studies have demonstrated beneficial effects, though others have not. Lithium has been shown to help with aggressiveness in children and adolescents in some studies.

Based on these sorts of studies on the effects of mood-stabilizing medications on behavioral problems, some child psychiatrists will prescribe a mood stabilizer to a patient whose mood syndrome is complicated by aggressive, irritable, impulsive behaviors, even if the classic bipolar symptoms don't seem to be present.

Combinations of medications in the treatment of severe mood disorders are becoming the rule rather than the exception. Almost by definition, early-onset mood disorders are severe mood disorders, and when the adolescent has a family history of bipolar disorder, it might be reasonable to add a mood stabilizer to his medication. How should the psychiatrist choose among the different mood stabilizers for a particular patient? It has been suggested that younger children seem to tolerate lithium better than older adolescents, because they are not as troubled by the weight gain and dermatological problems (remember that lithium can worsen acne). For older adolescents who may have more trouble with these side effects, valproate may be more appropriate, especially since these youngsters often have more problems with aggressiveness, which valproate has been shown to help.[42]

Even more so than with the antidepressants, the decision to add a mood stabilizer to an adolescent patient's medications and making a choice among the available mood-stabilizing medications is an art rather than a science. The published clinical studies on the use of these drugs for children and adolescents nearly always end with a sentence or two bemoaning the lack of research that proves the pattern of efficacy of these medications in young patients with mood disorders.

All this makes it very important that parents understand the target symptoms for which a mood stabilizer is being used, so they can help monitor their child for improvement, or lack of improvement, of these symptoms.

CHAPTER 8

Other Medications and Treatments

Although antidepressant and mood-stabilizing medications are the foundation for the treatment of depression and bipolar disorders, a variety of other medications are often used as adjunctive treatments. Sometimes these medications are used temporarily to relieve severe symptoms of irritability or anxiety, and sometimes they are an ongoing part of the patient's treatment.

ANTIPSYCHOTIC MEDICATIONS

A difficulty that immediately arises in discussing the antipsychotic medications is their unfortunate name. *Psychotic* is an imprecise term at best, and these medications have many more uses than simply treating psychotic symptoms. This group of medications has also been called the *major tranquilizers*, a label that perhaps more accurately describes the usefulness of these pharmaceuticals in the treatment of mood disorders. They can provide substantial and fast relief of the restlessness and mental anguish of severe depression and calm the agitation of mania.

First, though, a brief explanation about the word *psychosis* is in order. Psychosis can be thought of as a mental state or disorder in which a person's ability to comprehend the environment and react to it appropriately is severely impaired. The layperson's definition of *psychotic* might be "out of touch with reality." The person who is hearing voices (hallucinations) or who has bizarre idiosyncratic beliefs (delusions) is psychotic. The word also has a connotation of a severe disorganization of thinking and behavior, usually with restlessness and agitation. The manic syndrome is a good example of a state of psychosis, and I have already talked about "psychotic features" in depression.

In the 1930s, pharmaceutical compounds called *phenothiazines* were synthesized in Europe and were found to have antihistamine and sedative properties. One in particular, chlorpromazine, was found to be very useful in surgical anesthesia, because it deepened anesthetic sedation more safely than other available agents. In the early 1950s, two French psychiatrists carried out several clinical trials using chlorpromazine to treat highly agitated patients suffering from schizophrenia and mania. They noticed that in addition to its quieting and sleep-promoting effects, chlorpromazine made the hallucinations and bizarre delusional beliefs of many individuals with schizophrenia practically disappear. It also decreased the severity of the disorganization of thinking and agitated behavior seen in patients with acute mania. Chlorpromazine, in other words, had a *specific* effect on the cluster of symptoms usually referred to as "psychotic" symptoms, and thus the name for this group of drugs came about: *antipsychotic medications*. Occasionally, they are still referred to as *neuroleptic* medications (or *neuroleptics*), from *neuroleptique*, the French word coined from Greek roots that means, roughly, "affecting the nervous system." The term *major tranquilizers* was coined to distinguish these medications from *minor tranquilizers*, medications used for sleep problems and anxiety. But because these agents are much more than just "tranquilizers," this term has fallen out of favor too. The far-ranging effects of this group are more than simply "antipsychotic," but until a better term comes along, *antipsychotic medications* is what we're stuck with.

The main chemical effect of all the pharmaceuticals in this class is a blockade of dopamine receptors in the brain. In people with schizophrenia, neural circuits that use dopamine as their neurotransmitter may be dysfunctional in some way, and this may cause the bizarre hallucinations and disorders of thinking typical of that illness. Antipsychotics may work by affecting these systems in some as yet unknown way. Whether these medications alleviate the psychotic symptoms that sometimes complicate bipolar disorder in a similar fashion is as yet unknown.

After the development of the original group of antipsychotic medications, the phenothiazines, in the 1960s and 1970s several other potent dopamine-blocking medications were developed. The side-effect profile of

Table 8-1 Traditional Antipsychotic Medications

Generic Name	Brand Name
Chlorpromazine	Thorazine
Fluphenazine	Prolixin
Haloperidol	Haldol
Loxapine	Loxitane
Molindone	Moban
Perphenazine	Trilafon
Thioridazine	Mellaril
Thiothixene	Navane
Trifluoperazine	Stelazine

these newer medications was marginally better than that of the pheno-thiazines, but they did not represent much of an advance therapeutically.

More recently, several new antipsychotic medications have been introduced that not only have substantially fewer and less severe side effects but also are more effective for many patients. These agents are called "atypical antipsychotic medications" because although, like their predecessors, they block dopamine receptors (though not as potently), they differ from the typical antipsychotic medications in that they are also active at serotonin receptors. As you might guess, this effect is thought to explain why these medications might be more helpful in mood disorders.

Therapeutic Profile

A good number of clinical studies have reported on the safety and efficacy of these medications in the treatment of schizophrenia in young people. This is probably because symptoms of schizophrenia often begin in adolescence and because these medications are the foundation of medical treatment of this illness. There is much less clinical research, however, on the use of these medications in adolescents with mood disorders—even less than on the use of antidepressants and mood stabilizers. A 1999 article in the *Journal of the American Academy of Child and Adolescent Psychiatry*, titled "Antipsychotics in Children and Adolescents," does not even mention the use of these medications in young people for the treatment of mood disorders.[1]

Nevertheless, quite a few case reports and "open" medication trials have

Table 8-2 New Antipsychotic Medications

Generic Name	Brand Name
Clozapine	Clozaril
Olanzapine	Zyprexa
Quetiapine	Seroquel
Risperidone	Risperdal
Ziprasidone	Geodon

indicated that these medications are probably helpful in mood disorders. For example, a paper titled "Risperidone for Young Children with Mood Disorders and Aggressive Behaviors" reported the use of this medication in the treatment of a group of 5- to 16-year-olds with mood disorders who had "aggressive and violent behavior."[2] The authors found that two-thirds of these patients, who "had responded inadequately to several mood-stabilizing medications," had what was considered a "positive therapeutic response" to this atypical antipsychotic. This study also identified the most common reason for prescribing these medications in young people with mood disorders: for severe behavioral problems and poor response to other medication treatments. Also, while mood stabilizers and antidepressants take time to become effective, antipsychotic medications can reduce these symptoms quickly. In a young person with severe symptoms of irritability or aggressiveness who has never been on any medication, antipsychotic medications may be prescribed temporarily to reduce these symptoms until other medications have time to become effective.

Side Effects

The original antipsychotic medications have significant effects on muscle tone and movement, side effects caused by the dopamine blockade these agents cause. The newer agents do not cause these side-effect problems nearly as often, so they are now used much more frequently. In textbook discussions of these medications, you will see these problems referred to as *extrapyramidal symptoms,* or simply EPS. Dopamine is the main neurotransmitter in a complex circuit of brain areas called the *extrapyramidal system,* which coordinates movement. The term *extrapyramidal* contrasts this system with another brain system, called the *pyramidal* system because its main fibers are carried in triangular-shaped bundles into the spinal cord (the "spinal pyramids" or "pyramidal tract"). The pyramidal system controls the quick, accurate execution of fine muscle movement, and the extrapyramidal system makes sure that the rest of the body moves as needed for the smooth and graceful execution of these movements. Antipsychotic medications, by blocking the dopamine receptors in these extrapyramidal centers, can cause movements to become stiff and slow. *Acute dystonic reactions* are muscular spasms that usually involve the tongue and facial and neck muscles; they are more common in young male patients. People taking antipsychotic medications can also develop a very uncomfortable restlessness called *akathisia*, felt mostly in the legs. A person with akathisia often feels the need to walk or pace.

Fortunately, all these side effects are treatable, either by lowering the dose of medication or by adding one of several medications that are also used to treat Parkinson's disease. Although the side effects are uncomfortable, they are not dangerous and usually respond quickly to treatment.

People who took older antipsychotic medications over many years sometimes developed a side effect called *tardive dyskinesia* (TD). This consists of repetitive involuntary movements, usually of the facial muscles, usually chewing, blinking, or lip-pursing movements. There is no good treatment for TD other than discontinuing the medication. Because TD seemed to persist in some individuals even after they stopped taking the medication, it used to be thought that these problems were permanent. As it turns out, most TD symptoms *do* go away with time.

The great advantage of the newer antipsychotic medications is that most patients who take them have none of these extrapyramidal movement problems. Like the older agents, the newer ones can be sedating, especially at first, and are also associated with weight gain.

The first atypical antipsychotic, clozapine, was synthesized in laboratories in the 1960s but was not marketed in the United States until 1990. One of the reasons clozapine took so long to get on the market is that it causes a very dangerous drop in the number of white blood cells (a condition called *agranulocytosis*) in about 1 percent of patients.[3] This problem might have meant the end of the line for clozapine, were it not for the fact that it was found to be highly effective in treating patients with schizophrenia who derived no benefit from traditional antipsychotic medications. Dramatic case studies of patients with chronic treatment-resistant schizophrenia basically "awakening" from years of unrelenting psychotic symptoms after they started taking clozapine sustained the interest of clinicians and phar-

Table 8-3 Benzodiazepine Medications

Generic Name	Brand Name
Alprazolam	Xanax
Chlordiazepoxide	Librium
Clonazepam	Klonopin
Clorazepate	Tranxene
Diazepam	Valium
Lorazepam	Ativan

maceutical researchers in this medication. Following the discovery that the risk of agranulocytosis could be substantially reduced if the white blood cell count was monitored weekly, clozapine treatment became available to larger groups of patients.

None of the other atypical antipsychotics cause this problem, so weekly blood tests are not necessary with these medications.

BENZODIAZEPINES

The benzodiazepines, widely prescribed for severe anxiety and insomnia in adults, are probably best avoided in young people, except for very short-term use. These medications can be abused, and it's possible to become psychologically dependent on and even physically addicted to them. (Withdrawal symptoms in persons taking high doses of these medications can include very serious problems, including seizures.) Also, their sedating effects decrease over time, and after several weeks of use their effectiveness as tranquilizers decreases. For these reasons, benzodiazepines are best thought of as temporary measures.

ST. JOHN'S WORT

Hypericum perforatum, commonly known as St. John's wort, is one of about three hundred *Hypericum* species, shrubby perennial plants with bright yellow flowers that grow in most temperate regions of the world. Teas and other extracts of St. John's wort (often simply called hypericum) have been recommended by herbalists for centuries to treat everything from insomnia to the painful viral skin infection called shingles. In the late 1980s, hypericum was investigated as a possible treatment for HIV infection, when researchers discovered that it had activity against retroviruses—activity that, unfortunately, did not translate into clinical usefulness against HIV infection. Most of the scientific work so far on hypericum has been done in Germany, where there is intense interest in herbal medicine and herbal preparations are more widely available and, perhaps, are more seriously regarded as valid treatment options for serious illnesses. Several studies have compared hypericum extracts with placebo and with a standard antidepressant. The results of the earlier studies were generally quite encouraging, suggesting that hypericum extracts had an antidepressant effect that is clinically significant in some people. A 1996 article in the *British Medical Journal*, which systematically reviewed twenty-three different studies including a total of 1,757 patients, found that hypericum extracts "are more effective than placebo for the treatment of mild to moderately severe depressive disorders."[4] The review concluded that people taking hypericum preparations generally reported fewer and less severe side effects than those taking standard antidepressants.

But much work remains to be done to better understand which groups of patients will benefit from hypericum and which should be treated with better-established agents. Problems with the design of many of the original studies (all done on adults, by the way) have made it difficult to draw conclusions about the relative effectiveness of the two approaches. For example, in two studies comparing hypericum with the tricyclic antidepressants imipramine[5] and amitriptyline[6] in people with depression, the prescribed doses of the antidepressants in the studies were low—so low, in fact, that they would be considered ineffective by most psychiatrists.[7] Another problem is that these studies often lump together people with mild depression and people with more severe depression, making it difficult to know what kind(s) of depression hypericum is helpful for: mild depression, severe depression, or both.

One study that avoided all these problems tested St. John's wort against placebo in two hundred patients who had been rigorously evaluated and diagnosed with major depression. This study concluded that "the results do not support significant antidepressant or anti-anxiety effects for St. John's wort when compared to placebo in a clinical sample of depressed patients" and that "persons with major depression should not be treated with St. John's wort, given the morbidity and mortality risks of untreated or ineffectively treated major depression."[8] Thus, at present, it is difficult to recommend hypericum preparations for anyone with serious depression.

Some proponents of St. John's wort emphasize that it is a "natural" remedy and therefore inherently safer and better than "synthetic" pharmaceuticals. But it's important to understand that herbal preparations are *not* inherently safer than or superior to chemically synthesized compounds. Toxic substances such as nicotine and strychnine are found in plants, and some of the deadliest poisons we know of, the amatoxins, occur naturally in the "death cap" mushroom, *Amanita phalloides*.[9] Another important point: the lower incidence of side effects of herbal preparations can often be attributed to the lower concentration of the active compounds in these preparations, an advantage that is easily duplicated by using low doses of synthetic pharmaceutical.

Nevertheless, discovery of a pharmacologically active plant compound has often formed the basis for development of a much larger number of useful new drugs and led to other exciting discoveries. The chemical isolation of opium from the poppy plant led to the development of literally dozens of safer and more potent pain medications, and also to the discovery of similar compounds in the brain (called endorphins) — now the basis for an entire new branch of neurochemistry. As we learn more about hypericum, it may turn out that a whole new class of safer and more effective antidepressants will emerge derived from the active compounds found in St. John's wort.

OMEGA-3 FATTY ACIDS AND FISH OIL

There are a number of nutrients that we must consume in our diet, albeit in very small quantities, in order to remain healthy, compounds that our body cannot manufacture but that are nevertheless necessary for normal cellular functioning. The most familiar of these are, of course, vitamins, compounds manufactured by some plants and animals but not by humans. Their name, from the Latin word *vita* meaning "life," indicates just how important to health they are. Unless we eat foods that contain the vitamins we need, serious illness results. Scurvy, beriberi, and pellagra are three, now thankfully unfamiliar, illnesses that result from deficiencies of, respectively, vitamin C, vitamin B_1, and niacin. All these illnesses have significant central nervous system symptoms, especially B_1 deficiency, which causes severe central nervous system degeneration.

Another group of essential nutrients is the *essential fatty acids,* a collection of complex molecules found in some vegetables and other plant sources, but found in much larger amounts in most fish. Nutritionists have long touted the health benefits of diets rich in seafood, and the lower incidence of breast cancer and heart disease in the Japanese population has been attributed to a diet rich in seafood.

There is growing evidence that essential fatty acids, especially a subgroup called *omega-3 fatty acids*, may be useful in the treatment of mood disorders, especially bipolar disorder. The particular compounds thought to have the most health benefits have tongue-twisting names typical of complex organic compounds: eicosapentaenoic acid (EPA) and docosahexaenoic acid (DHA).

Several preliminary studies have indicated that omega-3 fatty acids, taken as fish oil capsules, are beneficial for individuals with mood disorders. A 1999 study showed that patients who took fish oil capsules in addition to their usual treatments for bipolar disorder had fewer relapses of mood symptoms over a period of four months than patients who took placebo capsules containing olive oil.[10] All subjects in this study were adults with bipolar I or II disorder, and all were taking a number of other medications during the study. Despite these limitations, the results are very exciting as they point to a whole new approach to the treatment of mood disorders with a new set of compounds. Other than very mild gastrointestinal discomfort and a fishy aftertaste, there are no significant side effects.

The possible mechanism of action of omega-3 fatty acids has been described. Studies show that these compounds are incorporated into cell membranes in association with molecules that are known to be involved in cell signaling. They seem to be active at some of the same points in cellular signaling mechanisms where lithium and valproate are thought to work. Given that valproate is, after all, a *synthetic* fatty acid, the idea that natural fatty acids might have benefits in mood disorders shouldn't seem strange at all.

Other circumstantial evidence has also been cited to support the importance of omega-3 fatty acids for good mental health. Archeological and epidemiological studies suggest that modern humans consume much less food rich in fatty acids than did ancient peoples and that, compared with our ancestors, we may be deficient in these important compounds. This fact, combined with the evidence that the prevalence of depression is increasing and the age of onset of mood disorders is decreasing, has been cited as further evidence of a link between these important compounds and mental health.[11]

The study referred to above used much higher doses of fish oil than are usually recommended by nutritionists, who also recommend eating more

Table 8-4 Omega-3 Fatty Acids in Fish

High in Omega-3 Fatty Acids
(more than 1,000 mg per serving)
  Salmon
  Tuna
  Trout
  Mackerel
  Anchovies
  Sardines
  Herring

Moderate in Omega-3 Fatty Acids
(500–900 mg per serving)
  Halibut
  Rockfish
  Swordfish
  Yellowfin tuna
  Whitefish
  Smelt
  Sea bass

Low in Omega-3 Fatty Acids
(less than 500 mg per serving)
  Catfish
  Shellfish: shrimp, crab, lobster
  Cod
  Flounder
  Mahi mahi
  Sea trout
  Perch

fish rather than taking capsules. Whether such a high dose of omega-3 fatty acids was a necessary element in the findings of the study is not known. A study that investigated the benefits of eating more fish high in omega-3 fatty acids for preventing stroke found an incremental benefit: the more fish the research subjects incorporated into their diet, the lower their risk of stroke became.[12]

Omega-3 fatty acid therapy is at this point an unproven treatment for mood disorders, so it should *not* be substituted for proven treatments. However, given the apparently low risk of these compounds, supplementation of standard treatments for mood disorders with fish oil capsules, under the supervision of the physician, may be an option some patients will want to explore.

ELECTROCONVULSIVE THERAPY

No survey of the available treatments of serious depression is complete without a discussion of electroconvulsive therapy, or ECT. A highly effective treatment for severe depression and also for both phases of bipolar disorder, ECT often provides dramatic and rapid relief of symptoms when other treatments have failed. Unfortunately, patients and their families resist this treatment because of myths and misconceptions about it. A review article titled "Half a Century of ECT Use in Young People" confirms the effectiveness of this treatment in children and adolescents, and the authors conclude that "serious complications [are] very rare."[13]

Too often, the popular media refer to ECT as "shock treatments," with all the unpleasant connotations of that term: *shock* defined as an unpleasant jolt or blow, or reminding one of the pain of an electric shock, such as the painful spark of static electricity that comes from touching a doorknob after crossing a carpeted room on a dry winter day. Calling ECT "shock treatments" is a bit like referring to modern surgery as "knife treatments"— accurate in a crude sort of way, but doing injustice to what is now a safe and effective treatment that can be literally life-saving.

Although the effectiveness of ECT in mood disorders was not a completely accidental discovery, the theory originally proposed to explain its benefit has been shown to have no validity, so the development of modern ECT was a kind of happy accident nonetheless. In the early 1930s, the Hungarian physician Joseph Ladislas von Meduna proposed that there was a mutual antagonism between epilepsy and schizophrenia: patients who suffered from epilepsy did not suffer from schizophrenia, and vice versa. Modern research has shown this is not the case, but von Meduna—convinced of this idea based on his examination of the microscopic appearance of the brain of persons with the two conditions—conducted animal experiments attempting to find a way to artificially produce seizure activity. In 1935, he published a paper reporting a dramatic symptom improvement following artificially induced seizures in several patients with schizophrenia. Von Meduna used injections to produce seizures, but several years later, two

Italian psychiatrists reported that seizures could be produced by briefly passing a low-voltage electrical current through the skull by means of electrodes applied to the scalp. Ugo Cerletti and Lucio Bini developed their technique in animals and then tried it on several patients with schizophrenia; they also reported remarkable success.

Although individuals with some forms of schizophrenia often did show improvement in some of their symptoms after these treatments, it quickly became apparent that severely depressed patients showed improvement that was little short of miraculous. With "electroshock" treatments, these patients had complete recovery from their symptoms within a matter of days.

One of the first articles to appear in the professional literature on ECT was a 1942 report on the treatment of two adolescents with ECT by two French psychiatrists. The following year, the same clinicians reported on a series of thirty youngsters with a variety of conditions who were treated with the new procedure. These physicians concluded that ECT was safe in this age group and was most effective in the treatment of "melancholia." Interest in ECT spread quickly around the globe.

Like many seemingly miraculous treatments, ECT was overprescribed at first and probably administered to many hundreds of persons whom it had little chance of helping. It's important to remember, however, that these were desperate times in psychiatry. With the discovery of antipsychotic medications nearly a decade away, and the discovery of antidepressants nearly two decades away, "little chance" of helping was better than no chance at all. Because ECT is a highly effective treatment for mania, some institutions were inclined to use it for any and all highly agitated patients, and sometimes on merely uncooperative ones. Another negative factor was that in the first decade or so after its development, ECT had very serious complications. An epileptic seizure is a violent event: all the muscles of the body contract simultaneously for a few moments, sometimes with such force that broken bones result. Also, breathing stops and heart rhythm irregularities can occur which can even be fatal.

The nearly indiscriminate overprescription of a therapy that had serious potential side effects led to a backlash against ECT. In the late 1960s and 1970s, although modern anesthetic techniques were making ECT safer and more careful research was being done to determine which psychiatric disorders the treatment helped with and which it did not, the damage to ECT's reputation was already done. (The film *One Flew over the Cuckoo's Nest*, awarded the Oscar for best movie in 1975, which depicted ECT as it would have been administered several decades earlier, certainly didn't help ECT's reputation.) State hospitals drew up regulations sharply curtailing its use, and legislation was in effect briefly in California banning the procedure. The prescription of ECT for young people was even more vigorously opposed, and even banned completely in several states for various groups of youngsters.

Fortunately for those who can benefit from ECT, the pendulum has swung back to center. Modern ECT is safer than most surgical procedures, side effects are minimal, and indications for its use have been clarified. A 1999 survey of twenty-six individuals who had received ECT before the age of 19 reported "the vast majority considered ECT a legitimate treatment and if medically indicated, would have ECT again and would recommend it to others."[14]

Modern ECT

Electroconvulsive therapy has been greatly improved by developments in anesthetic techniques. ECT is usually done in the recovery room of the surgical suite of a hospital, the area where surgical patients are taken for observation immediately following an operation. This location is used because ECT treatment is over in about sixty seconds, and most of the "treatment" time is actually the ten minutes or so it takes for the patient to awaken from general anesthesia. Some large psychiatric hospitals have their own treatment suites that are equipped like a recovery room.

Patients are usually hospitalized during a course of ECT, although, increasingly, ECT is given as an outpatient procedure, just like "same-day surgery." Sometimes a patient starts a course of ECT in the hospital and finishes it as an outpatient.

Electroconvulsive therapy is now done under general anesthesia just as safely as is surgery. Because each treatment lasts only a few minutes, intravenous barbiturate is used instead of the inhaled anesthetics used in most surgery. The crucial anesthetic advance for ECT was the introduction in the 1950s of agents called *muscle relaxants*, or more properly *neuromuscular blocking agents*. These medications, also given intravenously, temporarily paralyze the patient by blocking nervous center transmission to the muscles. This prevents the violent muscle contractions during seizures that characterized early ECT.

Immediately before the treatment, a patient usually receives an injection of a medication that prevents abnormal heart rhythms, an IV is started, and the patient is put to sleep with a barbiturate and then given the muscle relaxant. The patient is asleep and completely relaxed in less than five minutes. Electrode disks similar to those used to take cardiograms are applied to the scalp. Modern ECT equipment, designed specifically for this purpose, delivers a precisely timed and measured electrical stimulus: usually a half-second to several seconds in duration. In *bilateral* treatments, an electrode is applied over each temple; in *unilateral* treatments, where the object is to stimulate only half the brain, one electrode is placed in the middle of the forehead and the other at the temple. (Unilateral treatment causes less post-ECT confusion and memory problems—side effects discussed below—and is now used almost exclusively. Occasionally, unilateral treatments don't work as well, and some patients must therefore receive bilateral treatments.)

The "seizure" in modern ECT is pretty much an electrical event only, with few or none of the jerking movements that usually characterize seizures. Most ECT machines used today also record an electroencephalogram (a measurement of the electrical activity of the brain) through the same electrodes used to deliver the stimulus, so the physician can see how long the induced "seizure" lasts—usually twenty-five to forty-five seconds. A few brief muscle contractions might be observed during this time, but the muscle relaxant keeps the patient nearly motionless. There is usually a brief quickening of the heart rate and increase of blood pressure, which also signal that the "seizure" has occurred. The anesthetist applies a facemask breathing device to deliver oxygen to the patient until she wakes up five or ten minutes later and the treatment is over.

The only patients who absolutely can't receive ECT are those with medical conditions so severe that even ten to fifteen minutes of general anesthesia is too dangerous, for example, patients with severe cardiac or lung disease.

Typically, when the decision is made to give a course of ECT, most or even all psychiatric medications are stopped. (Sedative medications often shorten and otherwise interfere with the ECT "seizure," as do the antiepilepsy mood stabilizers. Lithium seems to make patients more prone to episodes of confusion after treatments.)

Patients awakening from anesthesia are a bit groggy, of course, and often are also slightly fuzzyheaded and feel "spacey" for another hour or so. This is probably related to the treatments themselves, not just the anesthesia, and resembles the mild postseizure confusion sometimes experienced by people with true epilepsy. Occasionally, a more severe period of confusion called delirium is seen, especially after bilateral treatments and especially towards the end of a course of treatments. Sedatives can treat this problem quickly, but when it occurs, consideration should be given to stopping the treatments or giving them less often.

The most troublesome possible side effects of ECT relate to its effect on memory; about two-thirds of patients report that ECT affects their memory in some way. The most common memory loss is for events occurring during the several weeks of the ECT treatments. Treatments are typically given three times a week and a patient typically needs six to twelve treatments for complete recovery, so a course of ECT will last two to four weeks. Patients not infrequently lose memory for some events that occurred during those weeks. Some also suffer *retrograde amnesia*: memory loss for a period of time before they started receiving ECT. This is thought to occur because ECT somehow disrupts the process by which shorter-term memories become incorporated into longer-term memory. (If you've ever lost an hour's worth of computer work because you didn't "save" your work before something untoward locked up your computer, you get the idea. The short-term memories that are still in the brain's memory "buffer" seem to be lost due to ECT.) Patients who have successfully completed a course of ECT may report not remembering checking into the hospital, or may not recollect a home visit or trip they took with their family during the treatments. This problem seems to be worst just after receiving ECT. In a study of forty-three patients interviewed about their memory a few weeks after completing ECT, some reported difficulty remembering events for a period of up to two years before their treatment. But when the subjects were tested again seven *months* after their treatment, these more distant memories were almost completely recovered.[15] One explanation for this finding is the known effect that severe depression has on memory. Several studies indicate that complaints of memory problems after ECT correlate better with the severity of patients' depression than with how they do on memory tests.[16] Unilateral ECT appears to sharply reduce the number of memory complaints.[17]

Data on the effect of ECT on memory in young people are scarcer, but one study of a group of adolescent patients who received ECT for bipolar disorder found that only 2 percent of them complained of any memory problems.[18] A more rigorous study of the longer-term effects of ECT on thinking and memory in adolescents—ten patients who had received ECT before the age of 19—involved testing learning ability and short-term memory and asking questions about their subjective sense of their memory ability. The testing was done an average of two years following the course of treatment. No differences were found in learning, short-term memory, or complaints about memory between the subjects who had received ECT and a similar group of subjects who had also been depressed but had never received ECT.[19]

The mechanism by which ECT works continues to be profoundly mysterious. During seizure activity, the neurons of the brain fire simultaneously and rhythmically and there is a massive discharge of many neurotransmitters. We used to compare ECT to cardiac defibrillation: just as applying a current to the heart can "reset" abnormal rhythms in cardiac muscle, perhaps ECT "resets" rhythmic discharges in the brain in some way. But newer work seems to indicate that, as with other treatments for bipolar disorder, the effect occurs at the level of the individual neurons. Animal experimentation indicates that ECT, like lithium, affects G proteins within the neurons. It may be that ECT, like lithium, works on the neuronal "tuning" mechanisms: the G protein–second messenger system discussed in chapter 5.

Prescription of ECT for Adolescents

Electroconvulsive therapy is perhaps the most effective treatment there is for severe depression and severe mania and often works more quickly than medications. Naturally, it should be a treatment consideration whenever a person continues to be severely depressed despite antidepressant medication treatment. It is *rapidly* effective: many patients have dramatic improvements after three or four treatments, that is, after five to seven days. Severely suicidal individuals, or those who have stopped eating and drinking and are in danger of malnutrition and dehydration—any patients for whom profound depression has become an imminently life-threatening illness—are candidates for ECT. For these individuals, the effectiveness of ECT can seem truly miraculous, as this account shows:

> On February 10, 1977, electroconvulsive treatment was administered for the first time to a 16-year-old female who had not eaten, spoken or walked unaided for the past four months . . . The first treatment produced an un-

clenching of the fists . . . The second treatment produced consumption of small amount of fluids . . . The fifth was productive of eating and talking normally . . . She was allowed to go home two days after the [seventh] treatment and for the past three months has been getting along nicely and doing all things previously done in a satisfactory fashion.[20]

Electroconvulsive therapy is also a highly effective treatment for mania. A 1994 review in the *American Journal of Psychiatry* of fifty years' experience of the use of ECT for treating mania found that it provided complete symptom remission or marked improvement in 80 percent of the manic patients studied. Many of the patients in these studies had failed to respond to many other available treatments—making this success rate all the more impressive.[21] ECT seems to work more quickly in mania than in depression. One study found that patients with mania recovered after an average of six treatments, about half the usual requirement for the treatment of depression.[22] Severely manic patients whose highly agitated state becomes physically dangerous are obviously candidates for ECT.

Although ECT can quickly interrupt an episode of depression or mania, the effect of the treatment doesn't usually last more than several months. Thus, medication treatment will still be necessary to sustain the benefit of ECT and keep the patient's mood state stable after the treatments are finished. Some experts are now recommending that medication be started before the treatments are finished. Depressed patients with bipolar disorder who receive ECT can become slightly hypomanic. Obviously, it's time to stop the treatments when this occurs. Unlike the antidepressants, however, ECT does not seem to increase the cycling of the illness.[23]

A survey of adolescents who had received ECT and of their parents, conducted in 2000, illustrates how difficult and frightening it is for parents to give consent for ECT for their children. Most of the parents volunteered, even before being asked by the researchers, that the decision was very difficult for them and the prospect of the treatment frightened them at the time they were asked to agree to it for their child. The use of electricity and the induction of seizures was the scariest part for them. But once the treatments were over, attitudes about them were positive. All the parents (and the adolescents too) said they thought ECT had been a helpful treatment that should be available to treat severe depression in young people.[24]

OTHER NEW TREATMENTS

Transcranial Stimulation

Repetitive transcranial magnetic stimulation (TMS, or sometimes rTMS) is a new experimental therapeutic technique, similar to ECT, that appears to be effective in treating mood disorders. TMS is currently a research technique only, but preliminary results are very encouraging. The great advantage of TMS over ECT is that TMS is much simpler to administer: no seizure activity is induced by the treatment and therefore no anesthesia is necessary.

This novel technique takes advantage of a principle of electromagnetism called *induction* (in which a magnetic field induces an electrical current in a nearby conductor) to deliver an electrical stimulus to the brain without applying electrical energy to the scalp (as in ECT). During TMS treatments, a magnetic coil is held against the scalp and the magnetic field that develops in the coil causes electrical current to flow through nearby neurons under the skull. No electricity passes through the skull as in ECT, only magnetic waves. Because the electrical current that is generated in the brain tissue by TMS is so small, a seizure does not occur—which is why no anesthesia is necessary. Pulses of magnetic energy are delivered over a period of about twenty minutes while the patient simply sits in a chair. The patient is awake and alert through the whole procedure. Other than some soreness from muscle stimulation, there appear to be no side effects of any kind.[25]

Transcranial magnetic stimulation has been used for a number of years to do brain mapping. Mapping of the motor areas of the brain involves stimulating a brain area and measuring for electrical activity in muscles controlled by that area. Stimulating sensory areas of the brain can cause a person to feel tingling in the part of the body that sends sensory messages to that brain area. Sophisticated TMS techniques are also being used to study language functions, as well as the organization of complex movements.

It is possible to give a placebo TMS treatment, allowing valid research on the efficacy of TMS in depression. (A true placebo-controlled study of ECT would mean giving two groups of patients anesthesia but giving the electrical stimulus only to patients in the experimental group. Risking anesthesia to receive a fake ECT treatment is something few people would volunteer for and, ethically, is a rather dubious idea.) When the TMS coil is applied to the scalp at a slightly different angle from that used to give treatments, it does not cause electrical current to flow through the brain tissue

Figure 8-1 Transcranial magnetic stimulation

and thus will not have the usual TMS effect. However, because the muscles are still stimulated, the slight muscle soreness associated with the treatment still occurs and research subjects have no way of knowing whether they are getting a sham treatment or the real thing. This makes the all-important double-blind placebo-controlled studies fairly easy to do.

Several studies indicate that the brain areas know as the left prefrontal lobes are less active than normal in depression. This finding has led researchers to try TMS treatments on depressed patients by stimulation of the left prefrontal lobes. Early results have been very promising. In one of the first studies on TMS in the treatment of depression, twelve patients received twenty TMS stimulations of two seconds each over a period of twenty minutes every weekday for two weeks.[26] Either before or after the two weeks of therapy, the subjects were given two weeks of "sham" treatments (the placebo), during which the TMS coil was held at an angle that would not cause brain tissue stimulation. The patients were tested for depressive symptoms by trained investigators using a standardized questionnaire. Neither the subject nor the investigator giving the mood questionnaire knew whether the patient was receiving real or sham TMS (making the study double blind). The study found statistically significant mood improvement after TMS treatments but not after the sham treatments. Several patients continued TMS after the completion of the study and experienced even further clinical improvement in their depressive symptoms. Another study found similar results in a group that included some individuals with bipolar disorder.[27] In several studies, patients with drug-resistant depression showed improvement after TMS.[28]

Transcranial magnetic stimulation is in its infancy. As of this writing, there are no published reports of its use in young people. All indications are that it will be safe, but its efficacy remains untested in this age range. The strength of the magnetic stimulation that is most beneficial, the exact placement of the coil, the number of treatments, and the duration of therapy are all under investigation at various centers around the world. Will TMS, like ECT, be effective in bipolar depression as well as in unipolar depression? How about in mania? These and many other questions remain to be answered. Perhaps the biggest unanswered question is: how does TMS work? It has always been thought that the seizure is the necessary therapeutic factor in ECT. Does TMS work in a different way? Or is it some kind of "gentler" ECT that works by a similar mechanism but without causing a seizure? (If the TMS coil is made to generate a strong enough magnetic field, a seizure can indeed be triggered with this technique, perhaps supporting the latter explanation.)

What is clear, however, is that TMS is a very promising development in the treatment of mood disorders and may open up a whole new array of treatment options.

Vagal Nerve Stimulation

Vagal nerve stimulation (VNS), another experimental approach for severe treatment-resistant depression, is also currently under investigation. Because it sometimes is discussed in the media, a brief description is in order. The vagal nerve (or *vagus*) is a long nerve that emerges from the base of the human brain and travels down the neck and into the chest and abdomen; it regulates a number of vital bodily functions such as digestion and heart rate. Its connections in the brain are through important centers thought to be involved in emotional regulation, and specifically mood regulation. VNS is done by means of a pacemaker-like device that must be surgically implanted to deliver the tiny electrical signals that stimulate the vagus.

Animal studies done as early as the 1930s demonstrated that electrical stimulation of the vagal nerve produced changes in the electrical activity of the brain. In the 1980s, it was demonstrated that VNS could control epileptic seizures in dogs. By the 1990s, VNS had become available for the treatment of intractable epilepsy in humans, first in Europe and then in the United States. And by the end of 2000, about six thousand patients worldwide had received VNS, almost all of them for the treatment of epilepsy. As with antiepilepsy medications that later turned out to be effective mood stabilizers, VNS was noted to have beneficial effects on mood in several of the patients who received it to treat their seizures. Several epilepsy patients had substantial antidepressant effects from VNS, even though the treatment didn't improve their seizure control.

In one of the first studies of VNS treatment in depression, thirty adults received VNS for severe, treatment-resistant depression; some of these patients had taken up to five different medications and received ECT, with little benefit. About half of the patients benefited from VNS.[29] This is still an experimental treatment, and, as of this writing, there are no reports of its use in young people.

CHAPTER 9

Counseling and Psychotherapy

Medical treatments such as pharmaceuticals often form the foundation of the treatment of serious mood disorders, but counseling and psychotherapy are important, perhaps indispensable, additional therapeutic interventions for these illnesses. Parents are often interested to know the answers to two very different questions about the treatment of depression with counseling and psychotherapy: first, whether this form of treatment is *necessary*, and, second, whether it is *sufficient*. Put another way, these questions become: "if medications are going to make the depression better, why bother with psychotherapy?" and "is it possible that psychotherapy alone will successfully treat depression and make medication treatment unnecessary?" I hope to persuade you that the "medication *versus* therapy" perspective is not a good way to think about the treatment of depression.

THE "BIOLOGY-PSYCHOLOGY" SPLIT IN PSYCHIATRY

In the early twentieth century, after the discovery of the biological causes of mental illnesses such as general paresis (central nervous system syphilis) and cretinism (mental retardation due to thyroid deficiency), psychiatric illnesses were divided into two categories: *organic* and *functional*. Organic psychiatric illnesses were "real" illnesses, caused by germs, or abnormal hormone levels, or something else that could be seen under a microscope or measured in a blood test. In functional illnesses, on the other hand, it was assumed that nothing was wrong with brain functioning, at least not in a physical sense. Patients with severe depression, manic-depressive illness, and even schizophrenia were having some kind of abnormal reaction to life events.

The question then became: why do some people have these very abnormal kinds of reactions while others do not? It was at this point that the attempt to understand and treat these illnesses turned away from medicine and towards psychology. Sigmund Freud spent his lifetime treating and trying to understand people who were unhappy in their relationships, disappointed in themselves for choices they had made, perhaps confused and anxious about life decisions they were facing. Freud and his followers developed a large and sophisticated system of understanding human behavior based on understanding childhood development. They developed the "talking treatment" for psychiatric problems: psychotherapy. This basically consisted of helping patients understand themselves better: let go of grudges, resentments, and fears triggered by traumatic experiences and learn better, more mature coping mechanisms. This approach has come to be called *dynamic* psychology or psychiatry and is based on the belief that mental life is best understood as a dynamic interplay between emotions and intellect, present circumstances and unconscious memories of past experiences, and many other psychological factors.

Although this approach was extremely successful in helping people with a wide variety of problems and symptoms, practitioners of dynamic psychotherapy soon discovered that it didn't make much of an impact on the symptoms of persons with major psychiatric illnesses such as schizophrenia or bipolar disorder. The explanation given was that these individuals were too disturbed or too immature or that their families were too dysfunctional for patients to benefit from therapy. Then a revolution occurred: imipramine, lithium, chlorpromazine, and other effective medications for "functional" illnesses were developed. Persons with depressive disorders, bipolar disorders, and schizophrenia and their families started leaving the therapists who often seemed to be blaming them for their illnesses for a new kind of doctor: the biological psychiatrist, the pharmacotherapist, someone who would treat them for a "real" illness.

For a time there was a kind of schism in American psychiatry between those who believed that dynamic psychology best explained mental illnesses and those who believed that biology was the key that would unlock the mysteries of psychiatric disorders.

In the mid-1970s, this biological psychiatry–dynamic psychiatry split was in full swing. Many departments of psychiatry in university medical centers proudly identified themselves as either "biological" or "psychodynamic" in their approach. Usually each camp denigrated the other: psychodynamic psychiatry was "touchy-feely" soft science based more on nineteenth-century literary theory than medicine; biological psychiatrists were "pill-pushers" who didn't even talk to their patients and had no appreciation for the human experience.

But a few departments of psychiatry taught their students and resident physicians that mental experiences were not just a series of chemical reactions or simply a collection of dynamically interrelated thoughts and feelings, but both. People with mood disorders are still people, still subject to disappointments and loss and relationship problems and blows to their self-esteem. To see their moods as just the expression of so many chemicals to be fine-tuned with more chemicals was to do them a great disservice. This schism has now healed for the most part, and even the most ardent biological psychiatrists understand that a psychodynamic understanding of the patient is *always* important.

Although there is certainly a place for dynamic psychotherapy in modern psychiatry—*including* traditional Freudian psychoanalysis and the psychoanalytic couch—the variety of available psychological treatments has broadened tremendously in the past twenty-five years or so. Sophisticated techniques have been developed that work for particular kinds of problems. Some involve individual sessions with a therapist, others a group setting. Some are very focused on a particular problem, such as family problems; some are symptom-focused, such as on depression or panic attacks; some are designed to last only a few sessions, others are more open ended. Some are not therapy in the traditional sense at all but are support groups made up of individuals who offer guidance and support to each other and don't even include a "therapist." Also, research is being done to determine which psychological treatments work best for which problems. The prescription of a certain kind of counseling or therapy for a particular kind of problem is often backed up by as much research as the prescription of a particular medication.

IS PSYCHOTHERAPY ALONE SUFFICIENT?

A number of reasonably well-designed clinical studies show that some forms of psychotherapy are by themselves effective treatments for many cases of adolescent depression. It's difficult, however, to decide from these studies *which* cases of adolescent depression can be successfully treated with psychotherapy alone. It seems clear from this work that psychotherapy alone is *not* very effective for the treatment of *severe* depression.

Some studies showing that psychotherapy is successful in treating adolescents with depression have recruited their research subjects from schools by means of screening questionnaires that identified students with symptoms of depression. Often, comparisons are made between a group of adolescents who receive treatment and a group who are put on a "waiting list," that is, are receiving no treatment at all. Given that it would be unethical to identify individuals with a serious medical problem and then not get them into treatment quickly, we can assume that the adolescents in many of these studies were, by and large, not very severely depressed.

Some studies have actually excluded severely depressed adolescents right up front. A 1996 study titled "A Controlled Trial of Brief Cognitive-Behavioral Intervention in Adolescent Patients with Depressive Disorders" (*cognitive-behavioral* therapy is a specific type of psychotherapy that I discuss later in this chapter) found that psychotherapy had a "clear advantage" in a group of depressed youngsters.[1] In this study, research subjects were chosen from individuals applying to an outpatient clinic specializing in adolescent depression. While this would suggest that a group of more seriously depressed youngsters was being studied, a closer reading of this paper reveals that any adolescent "taking or likely to require antidepressant medications" was excluded from the study.

Rather than focusing entirely on which patients psychotherapy can help, several studies of the treatment of adolescent depression with psychotherapy have tried to figure out why this treatment *doesn't* help some patients. A study in 2000 attempted to compare the efficacy of several different types of therapy in 12- to 18-year-olds with major depression.[2] It found that therapy was not very helpful for 21 percent of the adolescents who had been recruited into the study. These subjects had chronic depressive symptoms during 80 percent of the time the study was conducted—over a period of about two years. (This study had already eliminated more difficult to treat and severely ill patients by excluding adolescents with bipolar disorder, substance abuse, and other complicating factors.) The researchers reported that the subjects who did not respond to psychotherapy treatment had been assessed at the beginning of the study as being more severely depressed.

A study titled "Which Depressed Patients Respond to Cognitive-Behavioral Treatment?" also found that the nonresponders were the subjects who were more depressed at the beginning of the study.[3] This study also measured "impairment" in the subjects at the beginning of the treatment and found that adolescents who were having more trouble functioning in school and at home were less likely to benefit from psychotherapy. Perhaps the most interesting finding was that no particular pattern of individual symptoms predicted which subjects would benefit—that is, there weren't any "red flag" symptoms that seemed to predict that psychotherapy wouldn't work, symptoms such as suicidal thinking or significant weight loss. Subjects who had more symptoms and were functioning poorly didn't do as well with psychotherapy as did subjects with fewer symptoms who were functioning more normally. (This study had already excluded adolescents who were taking antidepressant medications.)

These studies would seem to indicate that psychotherapy alone can be sufficient to treat adolescents with less severe depression—but just what *less severe* is has not been defined very well. Clinical judgment and experience are still the requirements for successfully prescribing treatments for depression, whether medication or psychotherapy.

An important last note to add is that there is little doubt that psychotherapy alone is *never* sufficient to adequately treat bipolar disorder. Adolescents with bipolar disorder are uniformly excluded from such studies, and a large clinical literature on adults with bipolar disorders indicates that medication must always form the foundation of their treatment.

IS PSYCHOTHERAPY ALWAYS NECESSARY?

The related question of whether psychotherapy is always required for treating depressed adolescents is also an important one to try to answer. If medication is the more effective treatment for severe depression, why bother with time-consuming and expensive psychotherapy treatment? There is little research on adolescents to answer this question, but some studies in adults have tried to elucidate the issue. These have attempted to see whether combined treatment with medication and psychotherapy is more effective than either type of treatment alone. Many experts who have reviewed these studies conclude that there is sufficient evidence supporting the superiority of combination therapy to recommend this approach in official treatment guidelines.[4]

One of the problems with doing this kind of research, and also in making any specific recommendations, is that the term *psychotherapy* can cover a lot of territory. It might be helpful to stop for a moment and explore exactly what *psychotherapy* means. Dr. Jerome Frank, who spent his career researching the techniques and effectiveness of psychotherapy, defines it as any technique that attempts "to heal through persuasion" and characterizes the process as one of "employing measures to restore self-confidence and help [the patient] find more effective ways of mastering his problems." Frank emphasizes that psychotherapy works insofar as it can "clarify . . . symptoms and problems, inspire hopes, provide [the patient] with experiences of success or mastery, and stir him emotionally."[5]

Psychotherapy, then, is not just giving advice and encouragement (though these are certainly important constituents of the process); it also helps people to make sense of their negative feelings, understand the source of these feelings, and make the changes necessary to relieve them. Part education and part inspiration, psychotherapy tries to help the patient step outside herself and see her situation objectively, in order to identify changes in thinking and behavior that will make things better for her. Frank's research indicates that a crucial ingredient is the ability of the therapist to persuade the patient that things *can* get better.

MATCHING THE PSYCHOTHERAPY TO THE PATIENT

Different therapists use different theories to help their patients make sense of their situations. Freud and his followers emphasized a person's early childhood experiences as the most important issues, and other theories after Freud have focused on communication, changing thinking patterns, or family dynamics. The healing power of psychotherapy depends on the patient's being able to make use of new ways of thinking about his situation. This means that the type of therapy needs to be matched to the patient's problems and to his way of looking at them.

Cognitive-Behavioral Therapy

In the 1960s, Dr. Aaron Beck and his colleagues developed a theory of depression, and a psychotherapeutic treatment, called *cognitive therapy*.[6] This type of psychotherapy has been researched more thoroughly than most others and has a proven track record in helping with symptoms of depression; in some studies, it has been found to work as well as, or even better than, antidepressant medication for some patients.[7]

The theory of cognitive therapy maintains that people who are chronically or frequently depressed have developed a distorted view of themselves and of the world and have adopted certain patterns of thinking and reacting that perpetuate their problems. This emphasis on thinking, or *cognition*, lends the theory and the therapy their name. Research has shown that depressed adolescents tend to (1) think negatively about themselves, (2) interpret their experiences in a negative way, and (3) have a pessimistic view of the future. Cognitive theory calls this the "cognitive triad."[8]

The theory further proposes that all this negative thinking causes a person to develop a repertoire of mental habits called "schemas" or "negative automatic thoughts" that spring into action and reinforce the negative thinking.

▼
___

John is a 17-year-old high school junior whose application to enroll in a summer creative-writing seminar at the local university had just been turned down. He came to his therapy session and brought along a lengthy critique of the short story he had included with his application, a critique handwritten by the seminar's director, a well-known local author.

"You see, I should have known better than to apply for this seminar. Phillip Preston, no less, gives me the bad news. Now, I'm never going to be a writer."

"Why do you say that?" I asked.

"If someone like Preston thinks I can't write, I might as well give up. That's the last time I bother trying something I'm not cut out for."

"Did he say he thought you couldn't write?"

"Well, no, of course not."

"I see; this famous author and writing teacher doesn't tell his students what he thinks?"

"Well, no. That's not true. In fact, he's got a reputation for coming right out with his opinions to his students. He's supposed to be really tough but honest."

"But, he treats you differently from everyone else?"

John began to get a little annoyed. "Well, I wouldn't think so, but how should I know? I've never met the guy."

"What do you make of the fact that Professor Preston wrote to you himself?"

"Well, I did think it was unusual. My friend Ann just got a form letter with her rejection."

"Could it mean he was impressed with some aspects of your writing and wanted to encourage you?"

"He said the story was, quote-unquote, 'promising,'" John said a little sar-castically. "But I figured he was just being nice to a dumb kid."

"So, Professor Preston doesn't mean what he says?"

"But his comments were really negative," John went on glumly. "He went through the whole story, the plot line, the characters, everything, and shot them down one by one."

I continued to reinterpret John's negative take on everything: "He must have spent several hours with your story if he gave you back such a carefully detailed critique. Don't you think?"

"Yeah, I guess he wouldn't have taken all that time and trouble if he thought it was completely worthless. He told me to apply again next year, but—"

"But he was just being nice?"

John was quiet and seemed to be thinking hard.

I went on, "Didn't you tell me that juniors aren't usually accepted into this seminar?"

"Right," John said. "Mrs. Robinson had told me not to get my hopes up, that she'd never had a junior get accepted."

"So, this wasn't really such a surprise for either of you."

"Well, actually she seemed surprised. 'I thought you would be my first ju-nior to get accepted,' she said when I told her."

"But, she didn't mean it? Just being nice?"

John frowned.

"What did your Mrs. Robinson say when you showed her Preston's note."

"Well, I didn't show it to her. She told me to come by her office to discuss some of my other stories and applying next year, but I haven't yet."

"Because?"

John stopped talking and just the smallest hint of a smile appeared at the corners of his mouth. I went on, "Because Mrs. Robinson is being encourag-ing to you just to be nice?"

John nodded sheepishly. Then he asked, "Are you saying there's a pattern here?"

"What do you think?" I asked.

"You guys," he said, definitely smiling now. "You always answer a question with another question. Do they teach you that in therapist school?"

I couldn't resist: "What do *you* think?"

John is down on his talents and assumes everybody else is, too. In situa-tions that can be interpreted many different ways, both positive and negative, he tends to go for the negative rather than seek alternative, positive explanations. When something positive happens or is said to him, he ignores it or explains it away somehow (called *negative attributions*). This, in turn, causes him to do things that reinforce his negative thinking (like missing out on the support and encouragement his teacher obviously wants to give him when he comes to her office), and the vicious cycle repeats itself.

Cognitive-behavioral therapy is a very active form of therapy. Patients are asked to monitor and record their thinking and behavior patterns. There is an emphasis on diary keeping, and "homework" is often assigned. The therapist challenges the cognitive distortions and helps patients identify automatic negative thoughts and reinterpret events more positively. There is an emphasis on the here and now, not on the past, and patients are taught to modify behaviors and ways of thinking about themselves and what happens to them (a process called *cognitive restructuring*).

Cognitive-behavioral therapy is the best-studied type of psychotherapy for the treatment of depression in young people, and it has been proven effective in the treatment of less severe depression.

Interpersonal Psychotherapy

Interpersonal psychotherapy (IPT) is based on the premise that depression is best understood in the context of personal connections and that, regardless of its underlying causes, depression is always inextricably intertwined with the adolescent's interpersonal relationships. IPT does not assume that relationship problems *cause* depression, but it is thought that addressing relationship problems can alleviate depressive symptoms, regardless of the individual psychological or even biological contributions to depression. Originally developed to treat depression in adults, this type of therapy has been adapted for adolescents to focus better on the relationship issues common in this age group. IPT helps the adolescent deal with problematic or unsatisfying relationships and attempts to restructure relationships to make them more fulfilling.

Like cognitive-behavioral therapy, IPT is an active type of psychotherapy and focuses on the here and now, principally on enhancing communication in the adolescent's important relationships: with parents and peers and in dating relationships. IPT tries to help the adolescent learn a more open communication style and become better at listening to others. The therapist tries to help the adolescent become aware of his need to develop adult-like expectations of himself and an increased understanding of his parents' point of view. IPT works to clarify role expectations and addresses role disputes and transitions. By enhancing relationships and problem-solving skills, IPT helps strengthen the adolescent's peer and family relationships, providing an enhanced support system that he can turn to when negative things happen. It is thought that this helps the adolescent become more resilient and less likely to become depressed in the future.

In a study of 12- to 18-year-olds treated for depression with IPT for twelve weeks, patients reported a significant decrease in depressive symptoms and an improvement in their overall social functioning and functioning with friends and in dating relationships. They also reported improvement in their ability to think of alternative solutions to problems, to try them out, and then to use them to address difficulties.[9]

Family Therapy

There are many definitions of family therapy, but all types involve face-to-face work with multiple family members in order to focus on the interactions and dynamics of family relationships. The goal of family therapy for depressed adolescents is to decrease depressive symptoms and improve the adolescent's level of functioning by identifying and changing problems in the interactions within the family that may be responsible for initiating or exacerbating depression. As with interpersonal psychotherapy, there is less concern with the cause or causes of the depression than with current negative relationships among family members.

A depressed adolescent typically isolates herself from family members, and the irritability and disruptive behaviors that are often part of the picture of adolescent depression can poison family life. Situational stressors can cause a depressed adolescent to withdraw from family life and to rebuff the parental expressions of concern that her depressive behaviors then elicit. This rejection of parents' attempts to comfort and be helpful frustrates parents in turn, and they can then become angry and critical. This makes the adolescent more angry, guilty, and depressed. A vicious cycle of blame and hostility can start that becomes self-sustaining and very difficult to interrupt.

Family therapy tries to help the family reestablish constructive relationships by decreasing adolescent isolation and parental criticism and bolstering family cohesion. The therapist attempts to stimulate reattachment within the family by increasing trust and desire for parental love and support in the adolescent and by helping parents reestablish themselves in their roles as empathetic caregivers.

Often the therapist will attempt to reframe depression-related behavioral problems as symptomatic problems in family relationships rather than problems that emanate only from the depressed adolescent. This may involve understanding depressive behaviors as actually fulfilling a positive function within the family. (Mom and Dad are having problems in their relationship; Johnny is acting up because he thinks a crisis will bring the family closer together.) This often has the effect of absolving blame and shifting the family's focus from "whose fault is this?" to "how do we work together to make things better?"

Family therapists encourage all family members to get their feelings out in the open in constructive ways and to improve interpersonal communications. The therapist helps the family negotiate practical family issues such as curfew, chores, and dating, balancing the need for parental authority with the adolescent's need for increasing autonomy.

Because family therapy is so wide ranging and individualized to each family situation, it has been very difficult to do research on its effectiveness. Many studies have indicated, however, that family stresses and tensions predict relapse of depressive illnesses in adolescents. This suggests that family therapy will be very important when these kinds of tensions exist within the adolescent's family.

Insight-Oriented Psychotherapy

Insight-oriented psychotherapy (or "dynamic" psychotherapy) consists of individual meetings with a therapist, usually over an extended period of time (months or even years), in which the person in treatment discusses her past and present experiences and feelings with a goal of better self-understanding, acceptance, and personal growth. Disappointments and accomplishments, affections and enmities, fears, inspirations, passions, and worries—all are, as psychotherapists are fond of saying, "grist for the mill" of therapy. Patient and therapist will, of course, talk about such symptoms as sadness and anxiety as well, but insight-oriented psychotherapy tries to understand symptoms as signals that indicate underlying conflicts rather than as the focus of treatment in and of themselves. This more traditional type of psychotherapy emphasizes exploration of the *meaning* of symptoms and the development of self-awareness and maturity. More mature adolescents who have good communication skills, who are capable of the introspection and self-reflection that this type of treatment requires, and who are motivated to understand themselves better are more likely to benefit from insight-oriented therapy.

Dealing with psychological traumas and setbacks—past and present—that cause understandable feelings of sadness or anger or anxiety is a focus of insight-oriented psychotherapy, as are thinking patterns, self-attitudes, and interpersonal styles that disrupt a person's ability to be happy in relationships, effective in school or work, carefree in play, and confident about making decisions about the future. The complexity and subtlety of this kind of therapy is why psychotherapists often study and train in their profession for almost as many years as physicians do in theirs and why people are sometimes in therapy for months, even years, at a time. It is also why this kind of psychotherapy is such an intense, powerful experience and the therapeutic relationship between patient and therapist so unique.

Insight-oriented psychotherapy is often referred to as "open-ended" and can continue as long as the patient continues to feel that she is benefiting from it. The goals of treatment are very individual and can be quite far-ranging. For these reasons, efficacy research on this type of treatment has been nearly impossible to do.

Group Psychotherapy

Group therapy can be particularly helpful for adolescents, because they are often much more willing to talk about their feelings and difficulties to peers than to adults. Feedback and observations may have a much more powerful effect on an adolescent if coming from peers rather than from an adult therapist. In a group, young people can model and practice social skills and benefit from companionship and mutual support of same-age peers.

The therapist usually encourages group members to problem-solve for each other and give feedback and support to one another. Group members are helped to recognize feelings in themselves and others better, are coached on social problem-solving, and learn how to negotiate to resolve conflicts.

Group therapy is usually an adjunctive treatment to another type of psychotherapy rather than the sole treatment for depression, often to address a particular problem such as poor social skills. Substance-abuse treatment is frequently done in a group setting, where modeling of behaviors and role-playing exercises are very helpful for the adolescent to begin developing a substance-free coping and lifestyle. Group therapy helps youngsters see that others their own age have similar problems (sometimes *worse* problems) and helps them experience first-hand how peers successfully or unsuccessfully go about dealing with difficulties and setbacks.

CHOOSING A THERAPY AND A THERAPIST

Therapists rarely identify themselves as having a particular theoretical orientation or doing a particular kind of therapy. (One exception is that some therapists limit themselves to individual or to family therapy but do not do both.) This is probably just as well, as no one type of psychotherapy has been clearly proven to be superior to any other for the treatment of adolescent depression. Most therapists are, in fact, familiar with many psychotherapeutic techniques and will be able to adjust their therapeutic style based on their assessment of what will work best with a particular patient. A really good therapist will be able to shift back and forth as the therapy progresses, perhaps being more encouraging and directive when the adolescent is still very depressed and more passive, making the adolescent work harder, as he gets better.

Sometimes, it's not difficult to decide which psychotherapeutic technique has a good chance of being helpful for a depressed adolescent. The depressed youngster who tends to be self-blaming and too hard on himself or herself and whose depression is not complicated by disruptive behaviors or substance abuse might be a good candidate for a cognitive-behavioral approach. If the adolescent relates easily to adults and usually completes the kinds of homework assignments that this treatment orientation uses, so much the better. If the depressed adolescent's irritability and disruptive behaviors have resulted in such a toxic family atmosphere that family members can hardly speak to each other without arguing, family therapy would seem like a good place to begin. In chapter 13, I'll discuss dialectical-behavioral therapy (DBT), a special form of cognitive therapy that focuses on self-injurious ("cutting") behaviors. Sometimes during the course of treatment, complex issues are identified that call for the more in-depth approach that insight-oriented therapy provides. An adolescent who identifies a history of sexual trauma, for example, may need longer-term psychotherapy to deal with the complex issues that such a history raises, even after the depressive symptoms have abated.

Rather than seeking out a therapist with a particular theoretical orientation or type of training, it's important to find a therapist who is experienced in the treatment of adolescents and who is good at what she does. Usually, the treating psychiatrist will be familiar with good therapists in the community, as will pediatricians, school counselors, and clergy.

Remember: in addition to getting treatment for depression symptoms, the depressed adolescent usually needs treatment for the *consequences* of having been depressed. If a hospitalization has been necessary, the return to school may be quite difficult. The youngster will need to cope with the curiosity and possibly the cruelty of classmates and acquaintances, and will need help and support in formulating answers to their questions and responses to their teasing. Studies have indicated that peers often perceive the depressed adolescent as shyer and less popular than other children, and more apt to be teased by peers. A depressed adolescent may well have been an outcast and felt isolated for a long time, and usually needs help integrating back into his or her social situation, a situation that may have been somewhat uncomfortable for a long time.

Sometimes depressed adolescents have developed a dysfunctional peer group that they need to break away from. The youth may have developed relationships with younger, more immature children because of their poorer social skills, or peers who are substance abusers or who engage in delinquent behaviors. The adolescent recovering from depression will need considerable therapeutic support to be able to leave these dysfunctional but nevertheless comfortable relationships and develop relationships with healthier and more functional peers.

The adolescent will need to make peace with having a psychiatric illness and probably with taking medications and will need help in incorporating these experiences into his or her self-identity and coping with the stigmatization of psychiatric treatment. For all these reasons, psychotherapy is always an important component of the treatment of depression. Even if an adolescent has an excellent response to medications, he or she will need help dealing with all these sorts of issues.

THE PSYCHIATRIST-PSYCHOTHERAPIST: AN EXTINCT SPECIES?

You have probably noticed that throughout this chapter, I usually refer to the psychiatrist and the psychotherapist as two different individuals. Unfortunately, this has become more or less the rule rather than the exception in American psychiatry. It would, of course, be preferable for all sorts of reasons for the person prescribing medication and the person doing psychotherapy to be one and the same individual. But for a variety of complicated reasons, most adolescents with mood disorders will see a psychiatrist for medication management and a nonphysician therapist (often a social worker or psychologist) for therapy. Some of the reasons for this are the changes in medication management of mood disorders that have come about with the development of new medications: so many different pharmaceuticals are now used in psychiatry that staying skilled in their use has become increasingly time-consuming. Perhaps even more significantly, though, as more effective medications become available for more psychiatric problems, increasing numbers of people want to (and need to) see a psychiatrist for their treatment. There simply aren't enough psychiatrists to do medication management and therapy too, especially in busy clinics. Because medical school and psychiatric training take longer and cost more than the training required to become a psychotherapist, psychiatrists (especially those who specialize in treating children and adolescents) are usually more expensive than other professionals. When the administrator of a busy clinic or HMO is looking to staff a mental health program, "split" treatment (psychiatric treatment split between a psychiatrist for medication management and a nonphysician therapist for psychotherapy or counseling) means more cost-effective treatment for patients.

The superior cost-effectiveness of "split" treatment allows so many more patients to receive psychiatric treatment so much more cheaply that it's difficult to envision a return to the days when psychiatrists did therapy and prescribed medications too. Fortunately, there are excellent training programs for clinical social workers, psychologists, and counseling professionals that are producing superb psychotherapists. And as we have seen in this chapter, psychotherapy is becoming more specialized too. It has become nearly impossible to be both an expert therapist and an expert psychopharmacologist. For all of these reasons, two professionals rather than one will usually share the medication management and the therapy of the adolescent with a mood disorder.

PART III

Variations, Causes & Connections

In this group of chapters, I explore a number of related conditions and problems that frequently complicate the picture of adolescent depression. Chapter 10 addresses the complicated relationship between mood disorders and attention-deficit/hyperactivity disorder. ADHD is a common childhood diagnosis in adolescents who suffer from mood disorders, especially bipolar disorder. The links between these two problems are real, but also complex and controversial. I'll explain what ADHD is (and isn't) and introduce some of the controversies surrounding its diagnosis and treatment.

In chapter 11, I review alcoholism and substance abuse, looking at how these problems, for most people who suffer from them, are almost inextricably interwoven with mood disorders. This topic may well be the most important of the "connections" covered in this part of the book, because the problem of substance abuse is so common and also because it is the most dangerous. Numerous studies show that the combination of a mood disorder and substance abuse is a dangerous one. Individuals with both problems are at far greater risk of harming themselves with suicidal behavior.

Next comes a review of the symptoms, classification, and treatment of eating disorders. These mysterious illnesses are seen almost exclusively in young women, most of whom also suffer from a mood disorder. Anorexia nervosa is one of the deadliest of all psychiatric conditions, and its successful management requires vigorous and sustained treatment of both the disordered eating behaviors and the mood disorder that so frequently fuels and sustains them.

In chapter 13, I discuss "cutting," a complication of depression that is occurring with increasing frequency and seems in many ways surprisingly similar to substance abuse and some eating disorder symptoms. It is also frequently a manifestation of a mood disorder, but as with substance abuse and eating disorders, it requires specialized treatment in its own right. This chapter also takes up the topic of suicidal behavior among adolescents.

The last chapter in this part turns away from more clinical matters and towards a more scientific one, to a topic often of intense interest to adolescents with mood disorders and their families: the genetics of mood disorders.

CHAPTER 10

Attention-Deficit/ Hyperactivity Disorder

N o book on psychiatric problems in adolescents would be complete without a discussion of attention deficit/hyperactivity disorder (ADHD). Depending on whom you talk to, ADHD is either an undiagnosed epidemic, with thousands of young people going untreated, or an overblown fraud that has resulted in the needless prescribing of potentially addictive pharmaceuticals to a significant percentage of children and adolescents. As is usually the case with any issue that involves human behavior, the truth is more complicated, and neither of these extreme views seems to be quite correct. In this chapter, I discuss the diagnosis and treatment of ADHD and give you some idea of how this controversy has come about. I also discuss the relationship between ADHD and mood disorders.

WHAT IS ADHD?

In order to understand attention-deficit/hyperactivity disorder, it's useful to examine more closely what is meant by *attention*. Psychologists have conceptualized *attention* as requiring the following separate steps and processes:

1. Becoming aware of new information in the environment (the *stimulus*)
2. Beginning to process the detected information, and filtering out competing stimuli

3. Shifting attention when appropriate to the task at hand, while resisting the shifting of attention to nonessential stimuli
4. Organizing a response to the incoming information

It is important to note that the normal attention process involves focusing on some information in the environment and actively screening out other information. If you are making a presentation to a new client at her office and hear the siren of an emergency vehicle outside, you may pay attention to the siren for a moment, but you'll then shift your attention back to the business meeting. Chances are, if another vehicle sounding its siren goes by, you won't even be consciously aware of it. In some ways, this screening out of stimuli is the more important aspect of attention.

The other important concept to understand regarding ADHD is that of *executive function*. This set of brain functions, possibly unique to humans, involves self-control and behavioral regulation, suppression of impulses, and planning and sequencing of behaviors. The executive control center of the brain allows us to think about our situation and about what might happen in the future and to plan how we can influence what happens to us for the better. Executive functions mature as a child grows into an adult. These functions seem to be carried out in the frontal lobes of the cerebral cortex, the most advanced area of the human brain. We know that this area of the brain continues developing during adolescence, which seems to provide evidence that this area is where these mature types of brain functions are carried out. In addition to problems with attention, persons with ADHD have problems with executive function. This explains their impulsivity, or inability to plan well or delay gratification, and their tendency to overreact emotionally to stresses with angry outbursts.

A diagnosis of ADHD is considered when a child, adolescent, or adult has problems with level of attention or executive functioning that seem inconsistent with his age and expected level of maturity. The problem with making this diagnosis comes in deciding what is appropriate at any given age.

The first description of children for whom we would today make a diagnosis of ADHD was given in 1902 by British psychiatrist George Still, in a paper titled "Some Abnormal Psychical Conditions in Childhood."[1] Still described forty-three children with severe behavioral problems: aggressiveness, temper outbursts, defiance, and severe attention problems. Many of the children had epilepsy, mental retardation, or other evidence of brain damage of some kind. He suggested that these children had a "defect in moral control," meaning that they could not regulate their behavior normally. From the 1930s through the 1950s, psychiatrists emphasized the relationship between these problems and brain injuries of various types, whether actual brain trauma from accidents or damage from childhood brain infections such as sometime results from measles. At the same time, psychiatrists recognized that the behavioral and attention problems of these children resembled those of individuals who had suffered damage to their frontal lobes. The term *minimal brain damage* was coined to identify these cases. By the 1960s, it was recognized that many of the children and adolescents with these symptoms had no history of brain injury, so the term was changed to *minimal brain dysfunction* (MBD). More recently, the term *ADHD* has been used, to acknowledge that this problem may or may not be due to "brain dysfunction" and that the cause of the symptoms of ADHD is unknown.

For several decades now, the number of children and adolescents (and adults) whose problems are grouped under the ADHD umbrella has been growing significantly. Whereas the individuals given the predecessor diagnoses of ADHD were severely disturbed, often mentally retarded and brain-damaged children, today, adults with college degrees are being prescribed stimulant medication for ADHD because of concentration problems at work. Between 1990 and 1993, the quantity of the stimulant medication methylphenidate (Ritalin) manufactured in the United Sates nearly tripled, from about eighteen hundred to more than five thousand kilograms annually.[2] Are pediatricians and psychiatrists getting better at recognizing subtle cases of ADHD? Or are these medications being overprescribed? The jury remains out on this issue.

The difficulty in making the diagnosis of this disorder is that the behaviors that must be assessed occur along a continuum and are not abnormal in themselves: a level of attention and executive control that seems abnormal for a person of one age might be perfectly normal in someone younger. If, in the example of the business meeting given above, you interrupted your presentation by rushing over to the window every time an emergency vehicle went by, this would clearly not be age-appropriate behavior. But if a 4-year-old child were to do so, no one would be surprised or would consider the child's behavior abnormal. Children are more easily bored than adults and are more easily distracted by interesting and unusual stimuli in their environment. They become more able to focus as they get older.

Age is not the only variable that affects attention and executive functioning. Just as there is a range of body height and weight that is considered normal, brain functions vary among individuals within a range that can be considered normal. At all ages, people vary in their ability to concentrate and attend. When we use more common terms such as *patience* or *maturity* to describe some of the elements of executive function, it becomes obvious that people also vary in these qualities within a wide range of "normal."

So how does one decide how impulsive is too impulsive? Or how active is hyperactive? What amount of "fidgetiness" is normal for a 7-year-old boy? And how does one objectively measure it? The psychiatrist needs to answer these questions when considering a diagnosis of ADHD.

Simply giving an individual a trial of stimulant medication to see whether it helps cannot be used as a diagnostic tool, because stimulant medications will improve behavior in healthy children as well. Stimulants *always* help with attention and concentration. This is why they are so prone to be abused.

Although there are certainly children for whom the diagnosis of ADHD is difficult to make, other children have such severe problems with attention and executive functions that their behavior is very clearly outside the range of normal functioning. There is no doubt that these children have a disorder and need help. What is the clinical picture in these youngsters?

Children and adolescents with ADHD have great difficulty with sustaining attention and organizing themselves to complete tasks. These deficits result in delayed learning, poor study skills, and disruptive classroom behaviors. At younger ages, these problems may lead to poor grades, placement in special classes, and disciplinary suspension or even expulsion from school. Peers perceive a child with ADHD as irritating and immature (*executive functioning* is, after all, another term for what we often call *maturity*). Other children may exclude a child with ADHD from their activities, so his or her social skills can suffer. Peers learn quickly that it is easy to tease youngsters with ADHD and to set them up to get into trouble with adults. ADHD is not a benign disorder by any means, and aggressive treatment is necessary to prevent the sorts of problems these children encounter over time.

Attention-deficit/hyperactivity disorder persists into adolescence in about three-quarters of the children diagnosed with the condition. It interferes with school performance, self-esteem, and family relationships and predisposes teenagers to high-risk behaviors. Adolescents with ADHD have worse driving habits, more accidents, and more traffic tickets. They have first in-

Table 10-1 Stimulant Medications

Generic name	Brand name
Amphetamine/dextroamphetamine	Adderal
Dextroamphetamine	Dexedrine
Methylphenidate	Ritalin, Methylin, Concerta
Pemoline	Cylert

tercourse at an earlier age, more sexual partners, less use of birth control, more sexually transmitted diseases, and more teen pregnancies than their peers without ADHD.[3]

TREATMENT ISSUES

The safety and efficacy of stimulant medications for the treatment of children and adolescent with ADHD is one of the most studied areas in the field of psychiatry. In contrast to the small amount of research on the efficacy of most other psychiatric medications in children, more than 150 randomized controlled studies have been conducted on the use of stimulant medications in children and adolescents.

These studies indicate that stimulant medications improve attention and concentration and decrease impulsive behaviors such as fidgetiness and interrupting in the classroom, and also that these effects are sustained over time.

There is much less evidence that stimulant medications help with the behavioral "fall-out" of ADHD. Research data indicating that medication makes a difference for problems with academic performance, peer relationships, and social skills are scarce. For these reasons, it is important to realize that medication for ADHD is only part of a comprehensive treatment plan that should include interventions in the school (such as smaller class size, increased supervision, and sometimes specialized programs to enhance social skills). Counseling and psychotherapy and sometimes family education and therapy are also extremely important to address the many types of problems afflicting youngsters with ADHD.

MOOD DISORDERS AND ADHD

Psychiatrists use the term *co-morbidity* to describe two separate conditions or illnesses that frequently occur together in the same person. There is a high degree of co-morbidity between ADHD and mood disorders, in some studies as high as 75 percent.[4]

Children and young adolescents with bipolar disorder often do not have the discrete periods of elevated, usually euphoric mood seen in older adolescents and adults with this illness. Rather, they often have extreme irritability and prolonged aggressive temper tantrums called *affective storms*, and the abnormal mood is ongoing and continuous rather than episodic as in older individuals. Distractibility, impulsivity, hyperactivity, and "mood swings" are symptoms of both ADHD and mania. For these reasons, the diagnosis of both mood disorders and ADHD is difficult in young people, and the relationships between the two diagnoses are, at this point, still poorly understood.

The symptoms of ADHD and bipolar disorder can be differentiated in many youths, but some youngsters seem to have both disorders simultaneously. In one study of children already diagnosed with ADHD, 21 percent were also found to meet the diagnostic criteria for bipolar disorder by age 15. That is, they seemed to have both disorders. This suggests that, in some youngsters at least, ADHD symptoms may in fact be early signs of bipolar disorder. The children with ADHD who eventually developed bipolar symptoms had more severe symptoms and more disturbed behaviors. Even more of these children met the criteria for a diagnosis of major depression: 29 percent had major depression by age 11, and by age 15, 45 percent— nearly half—had been diagnosed with major depressive disorder.[5]

How do we understand the children whose ADHD seems to develop into bipolar disorder? Did they really have ADHD symptoms in the first place, or does very early onset bipolar disorder mimic ADHD in its early stages? Are ADHD and early-onset bipolar disorder two separate illnesses that share similar symptom pictures but have different causes? Can ADHD develop into bipolar disorder? Why? And what do we make of the extremely high co-morbidity between ADHD and mood disorder? The answers to these questions are not yet known, and the nature of the connection between ADHD and pediatric mood disorders is unclear.

It has been suggested that the link may be genetic. In studies that look at the family members of children with ADHD, the families are found to have high rates of mood disorders. Children of parents with mood disorders have high rates of ADHD. The researchers studying the group of young people with ADHD described above investigated the prevalence of mood disorder in the family members of these children. They found that relatives of children with ADHD and bipolar disorder were five times more likely to have bipolar disorder than were family members of children with only ADHD. They also found high rates of major depression among relatives of the children with ADHD and bipolar disorder. The researchers speculate that ADHD with bipolar disorder is a particular subtype of the illness.[6] Or, perhaps these are two separate illnesses that happen to be inherited together frequently because the genes that cause them are close to one another on the chromosome and are thus usually inherited together (more on chromosomes in chapter 14). The only certainty about this mysterious connection is that much research in the area remains to be done.

The practical issues raised by co-morbidity have to do with treatment. Specifically, if an adolescent has a combination of ADHD and a mood disorder, *both* will require treatment.

The combination of ADHD and bipolar disorder seems to be especially difficult to treat, and combinations of medications are often necessary. In a study of adolescents being treated for a manic episode with lithium, researchers compared treatment responses in adolescents with and without a history of childhood-onset ADHD. The adolescents with the ADHD history took significantly longer to get better during lithium treatment than did those with no history of ADHD symptoms. This appears to be further evidence that the combination of ADHD and bipolar disorder may be a subtype of illness and that it is especially challenging to treat.[7]

We know that stimulant medication can precipitate mania in patients with bipolar disorder. We know that early-onset depressions not uncommonly predict the development of mania and bipolar disorder later in adolescence. Therefore, the use of stimulant medications in depressed youngsters must be approached with extreme caution. Many clinicians recommend avoiding stimulant medications completely in young persons with bipolar disorders.

Although tricyclic antidepressant medications have not proved very helpful in the treatment of young people with depression, their efficacy in the treatment of ADHD is clearly proven. The newer antidepressant bupropion (Wellbutrin) has also been shown to be helpful. The problem here is the same as with stimulant medications: the possibility of precipitating mania in a predisposed youngster.

Clonidine (Catapres) and guanfacine (Tenex), medications used to treat high blood pressure in adults, have proved helpful in ADHD. Whereas stimulant medications help with inattention but are not very helpful for impulsivity and hyperactivity, clonidine and guanfacine seem to be effective in reducing these latter symptoms. There is also very preliminary evidence that medications that affect the neurotransmitter acetylcholine may be helpful for the symptoms of ADHD. Tacrine (Cognex) and donepezil (Aricept), two medications with this therapeutic mechanism that are used to treat Alzheimer's disease in the elderly, have been reported to be useful for the treatment of ADHD.[8]

CHAPTER 11

Alcohol and Drug Abuse

I n the last third of the twentieth century, young Americans achieved extraordinary levels of illicit drug use, either by historic comparisons in this country or by international comparisons with other countries."[1] As terrible as this assessment is for the health of American youth, the truth is that it has even more troubling implications for youngsters with serious depression and other mood disorders. We know from studies of adults that the combination of substance abuse and mood disorders is especially deadly: persons who have mood disorders and who also abuse alcohol or drugs have a greatly increased risk of completed suicide. Severe depression complicated by alcoholism or drug abuse has been found to be one of the most frequent diagnostic pictures in study after study on the psychiatric diagnoses of suicide victims. In a 1993 study, clinicians reviewed the medical records and interviewed the relatives of almost fourteen hundred adults who had died by suicide, in an attempt to make psychiatric diagnoses of the suicide victims. This study, which found that most of the suicide victims had suffered from a mood disorder, also found that *nearly half* (48 percent) had suffered from alcoholism or drug abuse.[2]

ADOLESCENT SUBSTANCE ABUSE

Surveys indicate that among adolescents, the number who try alcohol or drugs (substance *use*) is much higher than the number who use them regularly, which in turn is higher than the number who develop serious dependence and addiction problems. There are two important progressions that adolescents may move along as they develop substance-use problems. The first involves how often and how seriously they use, and the other involves which particular drugs they use.

The *stages of use* of adolescent drug use and abuse illustrate how the abused substance becomes a bigger and bigger part of the adolescent's mental life:

1. Curiosity or pre-abuse stage
   Does not use: opportunity for prevention
2. Experimentation stage
   Accepts alcohol or drugs from others
   May try drugs for fun and peer acceptance
   Does not usually show behavioral changes
3. Drug-seeking stage
   Seeks out a steadier supply of abused substance (either own
      supply or a peer group with easy access to substances)
   Needs more drugs to achieve the same feeling (tolerance)
   Uses more drugs, and more often, than planned
   Uses drugs more regularly to get high and escape reality
4. Drug-preoccupation stage
   Has a significant loss of control over drug use
   Has less regard for the consequences of drug use
   Develops legal and relationship problems
5. Addiction
   Finds drugs necessary to feel *normal*
   Uses drug daily, or even several times daily

As you will see later in the chapter, a number of factors determine how far along this continuum, and how quickly, an adolescent will progress. I'll jump the gun a little and tell you that depressed adolescents progress farther and faster than nondepressed adolescents.

The other type of progression is according to *substance type*, reflecting the use of increasingly "hard" drugs with increasingly severe health and legal consequences:

1. Drugs legal for adults
   Tobacco
   Alcohol

2. Less addictive drugs
    Marijuana
    Ecstasy and "club drugs"
3. More addictive drugs
    Cocaine
    Narcotics

There is no doubt that tobacco and alcohol are indeed "gateway" drugs that often precede the use of illicit and increasingly dangerous substances. A glance at the results of various surveys of adolescent drug use verifies the alarming progression some adolescents make along this continuum: one review of the subject noted that adolescent cigarette smokers were 16 times more likely to use alcohol and 11.4 times more likely to use illegal drugs than nonsmoking peers. Adolescents who used alcohol were 7.5 times more likely to use marijuana and 50 times more likely to experiment with cocaine than nondrinkers. Adolescents who smoked marijuana regularly were 104 times more likely to use cocaine.[3] The farther the adolescent moves along this continuum, the farther he or she is likely to go. It becomes apparent that even cigarette smoking puts some youngsters at the beginning of a rapid trajectory of drug use that can end in physical addiction to extremely dangerous substances.

Social factors such as patterns of use among peers and the availability of particular drugs in a particular community will affect a youth's entry into and movement through this continuum. Age factors are also relevant: "huffing," the inhalation of glue and paint fumes, for example, tends to be more of a problem in younger adolescents. Also, it is important not to regard *legal* substances as necessarily of low risk: more people die each year of tobacco-related illnesses than of any other substance-related illness. Alcohol-related illnesses and tobacco-related deaths far outnumber those due to any illegal drug. Nevertheless, increasing social impairment, legal consequences such as arrest and incarceration, and increasingly severe medical problems usually go hand in hand with the use of the "hard" drugs.

Adolescent drug abuse is a complex issue. A survey of all the substances that can be abused and the ramifications of their use for adolescents with mood disorders would require its own book. Therefore, in the following sections I cover only three substances likely to be abused: (1) alcohol, because it is the most widely abused substance, except for tobacco; (2) marijuana, because it is the most widely abused *illegal* substance; and (3) MDMA, or "ecstasy," because its rate of use by adolescents is rising very rapidly and because it has an undeserved reputation of being a "safe" high.

ALCOHOL ABUSE

Many medical definitions of alcoholism have been proposed over the years, and none of them involves the popular notions of what defines alcoholism: such behaviors as drinking alone or drinking before noon. Several decades of public education seem to have made most people aware that only a minority of persons with alcohol problems wind up as bleary-eyed panhandlers on downtown streets and that an alcoholic might well be able to hold down a job, pay taxes, and mow the lawn every Saturday morning. Fewer people realize, however, that an alcoholic can be someone who goes to high school and manages to maintain passing grades. As a recent article for pediatricians states, "Teenagers can and do become alcoholics."[4]

The National Council on Alcoholism and Drug Dependencies includes several factors in its definition of alcoholism: *impaired control over drinking, preoccupation with alcohol use, continued drinking in spite of adverse consequences*, and *denial*. The definition can just as easily be applied to any kind of substance abuse.

All definitions of problem drinking include a person's *loss of control* over drinking, perhaps the most important part of the definition. A teenager who drinks when alcohol is available even though he or she had made the decision not to is showing a loss of control over drinking. So is a young alcoholic who goes to a party intending to have one or two beers and ends up having seven or eight.

Preoccupation with alcohol means spending more and more time thinking about alcohol and about where and how to get it and how to drink without getting caught. Having availability of alcohol in mind when deciding which friends to hang out with and which parties to go to is a part of this preoccupation. Soon, alcohol is not just a part of social activities but rather the axis around which everything else revolves.

The alcoholic adolescent *continues to drink despite adverse consequences*, as alcohol begins to replace everything else as the most important thing in life and becomes the center of his world. No price is too high to pay to use it. Parental disapproval and punishment, falling grades, loss of friendships or privileges, even legal problems will not deter the alcoholic from his pursuit of alcohol.

Another important aspect of any definition of alcohol abuse (or any drug abuse) is alcoholics' *denial* of the seriousness of their problem with alcohol. The word *denial*, when used as a psychological term, means more than just a refutation or saying no. Rather, it is one of the many psychological *defense mechanisms* we all use to manage psychological conflicts and anxiety. Sigmund Freud originated the concept of defense mechanisms, and his daughter, the child therapist Anna Freud, elaborated upon his ideas about them. Sigmund Freud believed that a part of the mind he called the *ego* is constantly trying to balance conflicting demands that impinge upon it from within and without each individual. He called the ego's attempts to manage these conflicts *defense mechanisms* (or, more properly, *ego defense mechanisms.*) Denial, formulated as an immature way to manage psychological conflict, works by simply rejecting the very existence of one "side" of the conflict. The alcoholic who wants desperately to continue drinking and does not want to think of himself as a problem drinker (and thus have to *stop* drinking) deals with these opposing sets of desires by telling himself and everyone else that he does *not* have a drinking problem. It's important to emphasize that someone in denial truly *believes* that the thing he is denying is really *not true*. The alcoholic in denial *believes* that he does *not* have a drinking problem. When the teenage alcoholic says, "I can stop anytime I want to" or "I don't drink any more than my friends do," this is not simply making excuses for continuing with a behavior he knows is a problem. Rather, the problem drinker truly believes the things he tells others about his drinking.

Although alcohol is physically addicting and the withdrawal symptoms of abrupt cessation of heavy alcohol use are potentially fatal, a person can certainly have a drinking problem and not be *physically* addicted. Because adolescents do not have the degree of access to alcohol that adults do, true physical addiction to alcohol is less common in this age range. An important signal of physical addiction is a need to drink daily to prevent feeling "nervous" or "shaky." Persons with severe alcohol addiction also experience *blackouts*. These are episodes of memory loss that occur after a bout of heavy drinking. They may range from not remembering everything that happened at a party where the teenager became intoxicated to not remembering going to the party at all.

MARIJUANA ABUSE

For the quarter century or so that the National Institute on Drug Abuse has been surveying drug abuse among young people in the United States, marijuana has been the most widely used illicit drug. In 2000, 89 percent of high school seniors reported that they thought they could get marijuana either "very easily" or "fairly easily." More than three-quarters of tenth-grade students and nearly half of eighth-graders reported the same thing.

For many years, it was commonly believed that no one became physically addicted to marijuana and that it was therefore a comparatively "safe" drug to get high on. This is because cannabinoids, the active components of marijuana, are absorbed into the fat tissues during use and are slowly released when marijuana use stops, making for a sort of tapering off that often prevents withdrawal symptoms. Studies have demonstrated, however, that chronic marijuana users develop all the signs and symptoms of physical addiction. The main criteria for addiction are the development of *tolerance* to the effects of the drug and *withdrawal symptoms* when the drug use stops. In a study in which volunteers were given the same measured doses of cannabinoids daily for four weeks, the volunteers reported that the marijuana seemed to become "weaker" and their high was becoming progressively less intense, demonstrating their development of tolerance to the drug. A number of these volunteers became irritable and hostile and developed sleep problems after the drug was stopped.[5] Other studies have confirmed that persons who use marijuana regularly and then stop completely can develop anxiety and panic, depressed mood, irritability, loss of appetite, insomnia, and physical symptoms such as changes in heart rate and blood pressure, sweating, and diarrhea.

Because these effects develop several days after stopping the drug, users can convince themselves that they are only using the drug to "self-medicate" preexisting anxiety or depressive symptoms. A regular marijuana user might say she uses it to "calm her nerves," when in fact the use is to ward off the development of withdrawal symptoms.

Marijuana abusers have the same problems with loss of control as do alcoholics, becoming increasingly preoccupied with the drug and continuing to use it despite adverse consequences. A study at the University of Colorado surveyed more than two hundred adolescents who had been admitted to a substance-abuse facility because of problems with alcohol and other drugs. This is definitely a skewed population, but nevertheless the researchers had no trouble demonstrating the full-blown marijuana dependence syndrome: 97 percent of these youngsters had continued to use after realizing marijuana caused problems for them, and 85 percent reported that it interfered with home and school life or that they had been high in a situation where it was dangerous, such as driving. Smaller but still significant numbers reported that they had given up other activities to get or use marijuana and that they spent a great deal of their time getting, using, or getting over the effects of cannabis. Two-thirds of these youths reported withdrawal symptoms, and a quarter said they had used it before entering treatment in order to stop having withdrawal symptoms.[6] There's little doubt that for these youngsters, marijuana was a powerful and addicting drug whose grip on them had become unbreakable. As with alcohol, some individuals appear to use marijuana "socially" and maintain control over their use, but many do not. I will examine the factors that seem to help predict these differences a little later. Clearly, however, marijuana's reputation as a benign drug is undeserved.

"ECSTASY" AND "CLUB DRUGS"

Amphetamines include a group of compounds (of which methamphetamine is the most abused) that are potent stimulants of the central nervous system. "Speed," "crystal meth," and "ice" are street names for these pharmaceuticals. They make the user feel alert, energetic, and often elated. The user experiences increased initiative, motivation, and self-confidence, enhanced concentration, and often an increase in activities and productiveness without a need for sleep. Because both physical and mental performance are enhanced, these drugs are prone to be abused by athletes, students cramming for exams, long-distance drivers, and others who desire to artificially boost their alertness and performance. The effects are brief, however, and users often experience depression and fatigue after only a few hours of amphetamine use, which may require several days of recuperation. Longer-term use or binges of heavy use over several days usually cause a "crash" into more severe depression, with low mood, fatigue and lassitude, and loss of interest and pleasure in activities—the gamut of symptoms of a depressive illness. Changes in appetite also occur, as well as vivid, unpleasant dreams and other sleep disturbances that can take weeks to subside completely.

The parent compound, amphetamine, is one of the stimulant medications used to treat ADHD: amphetamine and the related compound dextroamphetamine are combined in the ADHD preparation Adderal; methylphenidate (Ritalin) is another stimulant medication. Diversion of these drugs from legitimate use is a source of some of the amphetamines used illicitly, but they are easily manufactured in basement laboratories from ephedrine, a related compound found in over-the-counter cold and allergy preparations, along with other fairly easily obtained chemical ingredients.

Recently, a group of amphetamine derivatives has started to eclipse the parent compounds in popularity, especially among young people. These substances are sometimes collectively referred to as "club drugs" or "designer drugs," and "ecstasy" is the most popular. The annual survey of adolescent drug use conducted by the National Institute on Drug Abuse noted a marked increase in the use of ecstasy in the late 1990s. Ecstasy is the compound MDMA (an abbreviation of its chemical name, 3,4-methylenedioxymethamphetamine), and a related compound is MDA (3,4-methylenedioxy-amphetamine). Although both are illegal now, these drugs were first synthesized in the 1910s by pharmaceutical companies as possible appetite suppressants. No therapeutic use for the compounds was ever discovered, and there was little interest in them until the 1970s, when MDA (called the "love drug" for a time) began to be illegally manufactured and widely abused, prompting the Federal Drug Enforcement Administration to declare MDA and MDMA illegal substances. Underground laboratories worked to make more powerful variations of these compounds, and in the process they produced compounds that were not covered under laws against the selling, distribution, and possession of illegal substances (hence the term *designer* drugs). By 2000, nearly two hundred of these drugs had been synthesized.[7] A pill that is called "ecstasy" may, in fact, be any one of these compounds.

Although MDMA is chemically derived from amphetamine, the molecule has structural similarities to mescaline and is often classified, like LSD, as a hallucinogen. Unlike LSD, MDMA does not usually cause hallucinations, but as with other drugs in this group, users report feeling that their emotions are deeper and more meaningful and that they achieve profound self-understanding and develop new perspectives and insights about themselves and their relationships. Intense sexual arousal is often noted as well (the reason, perhaps, why MDA was called the "love drug"). The amphetamine-like euphoria and confidence the drug produces makes these experiences all the more intense and powerful. The adverse psychological effects are, as might be expected, a combination of those reported to occur with amphetamines and hallucinogens: psychotic episodes, panic, and depression.

An individual's decision to use a particular drug is determined by a balance between the perceived benefits and perceived risks of using the drug. (This is truer prior to the development of dependence, after which cravings take on a life of their own and decision-making is impaired.) If the perceived benefits (such as the quality of the "high" and the other pleasurable effects the drug induces) outweigh the perceived risks (adverse physical and psychological reactions; the legal consequences of drug possession or distribution), the user will decide to use. The National Institute on Drug Abuse's annual survey of patterns of drug abuse among adolescents has noted that the abuse of "new" drugs spreads very quickly, because it takes only a few rumors and testimonials about the "benefits" to generate interest and willingness to experiment. It usually takes much longer for evidence of serious adverse effects to accumulate and even longer for this news to be disseminated. For an illustration of this pattern, one has only to think of the decade or so during which cocaine was touted as a harmless "party drug" and widely considered nonaddictive. MDMA and its derivatives seem to be in this "grace period" as the twenty-first century begins, unfortunately abetted (as the spread of misinformation about cocaine was abetted) by uncritical media. "Experiencing Ecstasy," an article published in January 2001 in the Sunday *New York Times*, reads in places like an enthusiastic endorsement of the drug and mentions very little of the rapidly accumulating evidence on the dangers of MDMA.

Increasingly seen in the psychiatric and toxicological literature are reports of a number of sudden deaths in users (the reasons for which are poorly understood), psychotic episodes, prolonged depressions, memory impairment, and thinking problems.

It seems that MDMA exerts its effects by potently altering the levels of serotonin in the brain. You might remember from chapter 6 that one of the groups of antidepressant medications has the effect of *boosting* serotonin levels in the brain. Serotonin seems to play a very important role in mood regulation, acting as a modulator for various brain circuits. MDMA (as well as other substances that cause a "high") seems to set off a kind of serotonin "storm" that results in intense pleasurable experiences. The aftermath of this storm is an "exhaustion" of the cells that produce serotonin and, consequently, a depletion of serotonin levels in the brain. This probably accounts for the symptoms of depression that follow MDMA use. A much more worrisome aftermath of MDMA use is suggested by experimental studies in rats and monkeys. The results demonstrate that MDMA actually destroys serotonin-producing neurons in the brain. The implication of this for human users is certainly not clear yet, but we know that there is a gradual loss of neurons as individuals age, a loss that is not usually significant because of the brain's excess capacity. But, if users of MDMA have depleted their "excess" serotonin neurons, killing them off by taking MDMA over a period of time, there is the possibility that psychiatric problems will emerge as these individuals age and progressively worsen as time goes on.[8]

MOOD DISORDERS AND SUBSTANCE ABUSE

Research indicates that adolescent drug *use* appears to be more closely related to a teen's social and peer factors, whereas substance *abuse* seems to be more closely related to biological and psychological factors. This is evident from looking at the numbers of adolescents who fall into "drug *use*" versus "drug *abuse*" categories in research surveys. The National Institute on Drug Abuse's annual survey of adolescent drug use for the year 2000 indicated that about 80 percent of high school seniors had drunk alcohol and 54 percent had used an illicit drug sometime in their lives. Data from other surveys suggest, however, that the number of adolescents with a substance-*abuse* problem, though large enough to be of grave concern, is significantly smaller, on the order of 10 percent.[9] In these studies, the biological and psychological factors associated with adolescent substance abuse are a family history of substance abuse (probably indicating a genetic predisposition) and a psychiatric diagnosis in the adolescent, the most common being ADHD and other behavioral problems and mood disorders. Studies also indicate that depressed adolescents are much more likely to progress from substance *use* to substance *abuse*.

Does having a mood disorder make adolescents more likely to use and abuse drugs and alcohol? Can alcoholism or drug abuse trigger the development of a mood disorder in someone who is genetically vulnerable? Do mood disorders and substance-abuse disorders have a common biochemical or genetic cause? There is some evidence to support an answer of yes to all three of these questions. Substance-abuse problems have been reported to precede the development of mood problems, to occur simultaneously, and to follow after them.

Several studies support the idea that depression puts youngsters at risk for the development of substance abuse. In one study, 76 percent of adolescents with substance-abuse problems who had been referred to a psychiatric clinic had depression problems, and in most of these youths, the psychological problems had *preceded* the substance-abuse problems, sometimes for up to a year.[10] This supports what has been called a "self-medicating" link between substance abuse and depression: the adolescent finds that alcohol or drugs numb the psychic pain of depression, at least temporarily. After a time, however, the substance abuse takes on a life of its own because of the powerful addictive potential of these chemicals. At this point, the depression and substance abuse, in effect, feed on each other. The adolescent drinks or uses drugs to get temporary relief from his feelings of depression, but since one of the after-effects of this "high" is a crash into worse depression, he uses again, and crashes again—and on and on the cycle spins, ever faster and more out of control.

Some studies have shown the development of alcohol and drug abuse preceding the development of mood disorders. The idea has been put forth that substance abuse somehow leads to depressive disorders. It's clear that alcohol and drug abuse adversely affect mood in the short run, especially stimulating drugs such as cocaine, amphetamines, and ecstasy. Perhaps ongoing use of drugs and alcohol can lead to more long-term problems with mood as well.

All abused substances appear to work by stimulating "reward" centers in the human brain. You have probably heard descriptions of experiments in which laboratory animals will push a lever that delivers an electrical stimulus to certain brain regions rather than push another one that delivers food to their cage, and will continue to do so until they're practically dead from hunger. When a similar lever device is used to deliver an intravenous dose of alcohol or another drug, the substances the laboratory animals will willingly and persistently self-administer in this way are almost exactly the same ones that humans use to get intoxicated: narcotics, cocaine, and certain stimulants and tranquilizers. And these are the same substances that humans abuse and become addicted to. Some drugs, including ecstasy and cocaine, affect these brain centers quickly and powerfully; others, such as marijuana, work more slowly, but they all work in the same way: by disrupting the normal operations of the brain's "feel good" circuitry. Perhaps repeated episodes of drug use disrupt this circuitry in more profound and long-lasting ways and a mood disorder is the result. (Remember that animal studies have demonstrated that MDMA kills serotonin neurons in the brain.)

Finally, it may be that similar biological and psychological factors underlie the development of *both* mood disorders and substance-abuse disorders and that both types of problems are better thought of as two sides of the same coin.

TREATMENT ISSUES

Numerous clinical studies have shown a strong connection between adolescent substance use and adolescent mood disorders. One study followed up on a group of about seven hundred youngsters for approximately nine years to examine the relationship between substance use and depression. Not surprisingly, it found that depressed youngsters were more likely to use drugs and alcohol. It also found a roughly linear correlation between depression and drug use: the rate of depression problems went up in proportion to the severity of substance use. Put another way, the more severe the substance-use problem, the more likely the adolescent was to be suffering from a depressive disorder.[11]

But what about the question of whether one type of disorder *causes* the other? This question has important ramifications for treating these problems in individuals. If the "self-medication" hypothesis is true and depressed adolescents use alcohol and drugs in an attempt to "treat" their depressed feelings, this would suggest that successful treatment of the mood disorder should make the substance-abuse problem simply go away on its own. If the substance abuse is causing the mood disorder, then remaining abstinent from the abused substances should make the mood disorder go away. There are research studies to support both scenarios, which probably means that both can occur.

I think most psychiatrists who treat mood disorders have seen both of these scenarios in patients, and most would agree that when a mood disorder and a substance-abuse problem occur together, they are best thought of as two problems that *both* need aggressive treatment. Either of these problems can precede and seem to trigger the other, which then takes on a life of its own and therefore requires treatment of its own as well. In my own experience, patients who do not get treatment for both problems will not recover from either.

The first goal of treatment for substance abuse is to interrupt the drinking or drug use. Admission to a psychiatric hospital or other treatment facility is often necessary to remove the adolescent from an environment where he or she can still obtain and use alcohol or drugs. Family involvement is very important for treatment to be successful, by improving communication among family members and helping parents to provide guidance and set limits with the adolescent.

Studies of adult alcoholics and cocaine abusers have shown that regular use of intoxicating substances alters brain functioning. Specifically, functioning is disrupted in the prefrontal cortex, an area of the brain thought to be involved in the "executive functions" such as self-control, delay of gratification, and inhibition of impulses (as I discussed in chapter 10). Studies of brain metabolism show that only after many *months* of sobriety are these brain areas functioning normally again.[12] During this time, the recovering substance abuser is still at grave risk of relapse. The treatment of substance-abuse problems must therefore be a long-term commitment. A brief "detox" admission to a hospital or several weeks of intensive outpatient treatment is not sufficient to have a long-lasting impact on substance abuse in an adolescent who has progressed beyond the "experimentation" stage of alcohol or drug use.

Although alcohol and drug use may stop for several months after intensive treatment, many studies have shown that abstinence does not last if the youth doesn't get maintenance treatment of some kind. According to one study of the treatment of adolescent drug abuse based on the twelve-step program of Alcoholics Anonymous, just as many adolescents who had completed a short-term treatment program relapsed by the twelve-month mark as those who hadn't even completed the program.[13] Often the adolescent needs help in developing an alcohol-free and drug-free lifestyle and in making some necessary major changes in his or her peer group and recreational activities, changes that the adolescent can make only with time, counseling, and support.

Some youngsters can move from a hospitalization or detoxification program of several days'—or weeks'—duration to outpatient care. This is often possible if the adolescent's functioning level was not too severely affected by drug use and it's possible to move back into school and family life fairly easily. If drinking and drug use have reduced the adolescent's life to shambles, however, longer-term residential treatment will be necessary.

Youths who have dropped out of or been suspended from school, or who have developed run-away and other disruptive behaviors that make return-ing to live with the family tense and difficult, will probably need the struc-tured rehabilitation of a residential or "half-way house" setting. These ado-lescents require the professional supervision and guidance, structure, and support provided in these settings to make the changes in behavioral pat-terns necessary to maintain their sobriety.

Adolescents who abuse alcohol and drugs to any substantial degree es-sentially stop the process of psychological maturation. Their emotional de-velopment is arrested at the point where they started using substances heav-ily. An 18-year-old who has been smoking marijuana regularly for two or three years may have the emotional maturity of a 15-year-old and will lack the more mature coping, problem-solving, and communication skills ex-pected for his or her chronological age. When this adolescent gets "clean," parents may be disappointed that their child seems to be immature for his or her age and compared with same-age peers. The adolescent may find it difficult to feel comfortable with same-age peers. For all these reasons, counseling and psychotherapy, including family therapy, are often neces-sary and extremely beneficial for all involved. I'll be discussing how to cope better with substance-abuse issues in the family in chapter 16.

CHAPTER 12

Eating Disorders

E ating disorders are a group of psychiatric syndromes that share the common element of a distortion of normal eating behaviors. Individuals with an eating disorder may eat too little or too much, but they all share a preoccupation with food, calories, and weight that comes to be all-engrossing and pathological, often with dangerous, sometimes even deadly, consequences. Eating disorders are predominantly disorders of adolescent girls, and most of these individuals have mood disorders as well.

▼

Jennifer had only blacked out for a moment, it seemed, but she was still glassy-eyed and quiet when the ambulance arrived. The phys ed teacher had whisked horrified friends out of the gym and called the school nurse, Mrs. Coleman, who found Jennifer's pulse to be alarmingly low and was having trouble taking her blood pressure. When Mrs. Coleman hiked up the sleeve of the girl's sweatshirt to take her blood pressure, she was taken aback by how skinny Jennifer's arm was.

"Has this girl been sick?" she asked.

"Not that I know of," replied the teacher. "At least not anything serious, I don't think. She's missed a few days here and there, but that's all."

They heard the sirens wailing up the school driveway. Good, thought Mrs. Coleman, they're here.

She looked down at Jennifer again. "Why are you wearing these heavy sweats in June?" she asked. Perhaps the girl had become overheated and fainted.

"I'm always cold," replied Jennifer listlessly.

The gymnasium doors clanged open and three paramedics in sharply pressed blues briskly walked in. Mrs. Coleman and the teacher stood back, and Jennifer was on the gurney in seconds. One of the paramedics pumped up the blood pressure cuff that was still on the girl's arm and listened intently with her stethoscope. "Sixty-five over forty," she gasped. Another paramedic had already pricked Jennifer's finger and squeezed a drop of blood into what looked like a hand-held calculator. He read the number that glowed on its little screen. "Her blood glucose is only thirty-seven, Kate." Kate looked down at Jennifer. "Are you diabetic, honey? Do you take insulin?" Jennifer shook her head weakly.

"What did you have for breakfast today, sweetie?"

"A vitamin pill."

"We're going to start an IV on you, Jennifer." In a moment, Jennifer, the gurney, and the three paramedics were moving towards the door. "Tell her parents we're taking her to Memorial. We'll need them to sign for treatment." The gymnasium doors clanged shut. As the echoes of the door's banging died away, the siren's wail started up, and then faded.

Mrs. Coleman turned to the teacher. "Has this student seemed tired to you lately? Has she had trouble keeping up with the others in this class?"

"No. Jennifer's always full of energy. But this isn't really a class; it's an aerobics group for junior girls with weight problems. Participation is voluntary."

"Weight problems?" Mrs. Coleman said. "Carol, that girl does *not* have a weight problem."

"I started the group last month and Jennifer was the first to sign up. I didn't think she looked overweight, but it's hard to tell with those baggy clothes she always wears."

Mrs. Coleman looked thoughtful for a moment, and then asked, "Do you ask these girls how much weight they want to lose when they sign up?"

"They fill out a form with their current weight and their goal weight. I remember that Jennifer left those questions blank. I just thought she was embarrassed—"

Mrs. Coleman wasn't listening anymore, though. She realized that this girl probably *did* have a weight problem, but not the kind of problem an aerobics class would help with. When she spoke with Jennifer's mother on the phone, she asked about the girl's eating habits.

"They're terrible. I know she's too skinny. But she won't eat with us anymore. I almost think it's better that way because every meal turned into a screaming match. We can't even talk about it around here. Her father gets so mad about it that I worry about his blood pressure getting out of control again."

"Mrs. Andrews," the nurse said slowly, "I think Jennifer might have an eating disorder."

By the time pop singer Karen Carpenter died of anorexia nervosa in 1983—an event that brought eating disorders to the consciousness of most Americans for the first time—physicians had been aware of this mysterious group of psychiatric illnesses for more than two centuries. A Dr. R. Morton wrote in a 1694 treatise on "consumptions" (an old word for any illness characterized by physical wasting away) of "a nervous atrophy . . . a wasting of the body without any remarkable fever, cough, or shortness of breath" that he attributed to a "distemper'd state of the brain." In 1874, the English physician William Withey Gull coined the term *anorexia nervosa* to describe "a morbid mental state" that resulted in extreme weight loss. Gull realized that the weight loss was not due to a bodily illness like tuberculosis or an intestinal disease but was instead the result of "simple starvation."

But it was the French alienist (*alienist* is a nineteenth-century term for a psychiatrist) Lasègue who first captured the essential elements of this form of the illness: a "refusal of food" that becomes "the sole object of preoccupation and conversation" such that "the circle within which revolve the ideas and sentiments of the patient becomes more narrowed." Lasègue described the disconnect between the patient's appearance and her perception of her appearance and her assessment of her nutritional needs: "The patient, when told that she cannot live upon an amount of food that would not support a young infant, replies that it furnishes sufficient nourishment for her, adding that she is neither changed nor thinner." Lasègue also recognized the upheaval the syndrome causes in families and the frustration and powerlessness of the parents of these patients. He noted that the family "has but two methods at its service which it always exhausts—entreaties and menaces."[1]

In the 1980s, it was increasingly recognized that self-starvation is not the only serious abnormal eating syndrome. Also described were individuals, often of normal weight, who binged on huge amounts of food in a matter of hours or even minutes and then caused themselves to vomit what they had eaten . The terms *binge-purge syndrome* and *bulimia nervosa* (or simply *bulimia*) were coined to describe this condition.

More recently, descriptions have appeared in the psychiatric literature of overweight patients who binge but do not induce vomiting or use other means to compensate for their increased calorie intake, and the diagnosis *binge-eating disorder* has been proposed to designate this syndrome.

It has been suggested that perhaps the biggest group of persons with abnormal eating behaviors does not fit neatly into any one of these classifications; these individuals have elements of several eating disorders or shift from one clinical picture to another over time. Abnormal eating syndromes cover a wide range of problems, from those posing only minor risks to health to those that are life-threatening.

As with adolescent substance abuse, the topic of eating disorders is an enormous and complex one that could easily fill a book of its own. What follows, then, is a brief overview of the main symptoms of the disorders, just to introduce them and to make it easier to understand the interplay between these syndromes and the mood disorders.

ANOREXIA NERVOSA

The most dramatic and severe of the eating disorders is anorexia nervosa. People with this disorder believe they are overweight, even obese, and restrict their food intake to lose weight. They lose their objectivity about calories, weight, and appearance, and they continue to think they are overweight despite the emaciated appearance of their bodies. Their drive to lose weight takes on a life of its own, and despite their steadily decreasing weight, they continue trying to lose even more. The syndrome is, in a sense, incorrectly named, because the word *anorexia*, a medical term for "loss of appetite," does *not* characterize these individuals (except perhaps in the advanced stages of starvation, when their brain functions are abnormal in many different ways). People with anorexia do not lose their appetite but rather *fight* their hunger and, after a time, the struggle against their appetite becomes an end in itself, the focus of all their energies.

Often, the individual starts out with a desire to lose what might indeed be extra pounds, but then she cannot identify or be satisfied with a healthy goal weight. She may identify an initial goal weight of, say, 110 pounds, but after reaching this initial goal decides to get down to 105. At 105 pounds, the new goal becomes 100, then 95, and eventually the only goal is to weigh less than the day before—with no end in sight. She becomes convinced that if she starts to gain weight she will lose control of her eating and her ability to maintain her weight and will become enormously obese. In other cases, the person realizes she is thin, but nevertheless worries that some part of her body, such as her abdomen or buttocks, is "fat." Either way, eating comes to be viewed as a vice; taking needed nourishment is "giving in."

As others notice the girl's increasing thinness with alarm, eating and meals become more and more tense. As Lasègue observed in the families of his patients, "the delicacies of the table are multiplied in the hope of stimulating the appetite; but the more the solicitude increases, the more the appetite diminishes. The patient disdainfully tastes the new [foods] and after having thus shown her willingness, holds herself absolved from obligation to do more."

Anorectic individuals not only fast but also exercise excessively in order to lose weight. They may use laxatives and diuretics (fluid pills) to decrease calories and weight. And to avoid the stares and comments of others, they dress in baggy clothing that conceals their emaciation.

Eventually, the physical consequences of starvation begin to take their toll. Menstruation stops, heart rate slows, and hands and feet become cold as the body attempts to conserve calories. Skin becomes dry, the hair may fall out, and the person complains of fatigue and is noted to be listless and lethargic. Dizzy spells and fainting occur. Eventually, sodium and potassium imbalances affect cellular functions, heart rhythm abnormalities develop, and the girl can die from cardiac arrest.

The treatment of anorexia nervosa focuses on refeeding the patient in order to reverse the distortions in thinking that are due to starvation. Then, a lengthy retraining process must occur during which the patient relearns normal eating patterns and changes her feelings about herself, her weight, and her relationship with food and calories. In severe cases, lengthy psychiatric hospitalization is necessary to accomplish this work.

BULIMIA NERVOSA

The hallmark of bulimia nervosa is binge eating, during which the individual eats an enormous amount of food, often sweet high-calorie foods, over a period of an hour or so. She may eat an entire gallon of ice cream at one sitting, dozens of donuts, pizzas by the carton, candy by the pound, usually stopping only when physically incapable of taking in any more food. A binge is a private affair undertaken secretly and alone; the food consumption is frenzied, joyless, and obsessive, and the bulimic feels out of control, almost "out of body," while it is happening.

When she cannot force another bite, the bulimic is overcome with disgust and shame at what she has done and seeks a way to rid herself of the calorie load. The vast majority of people with bulimia do this by forcing themselves to vomit. This provides them relief from the physical discomfort brought on by the binge and also reduces their fear of gaining weight from such an enormous intake of calories. In the early stages of the disorder, individuals with bulimia usually stimulate their gag reflex by putting a finger or spoon down the throat, but later in the course of the disorder they often become adept at vomiting at will. Those who do not manage this may actually develop a callus on the first knuckle of their finger from the repeated abrasions caused by their teeth during self-stimulation to induce vomiting. Individuals with bulimia also misuse laxatives and diuretics to get rid of calories and water-weight.

The binge is often an unplanned and impulsive response to some uncomfortable emotional state. Like those with anorexia nervosa, these girls and young women are abnormally preoccupied with their weight and body image and, outside their binges, are often strictly controlling their diet and avoiding high-calorie foods.

Individuals with bulimia nervosa are usually impulsive in other areas of their lives, and they often have a history of substance abuse, self-mutilation, and suicide attempts. Many anorectics also have bulimic behaviors, and approximately 40 percent of them have a more prolonged bulimic phase in the course of their illness or recovery.[2]

Most individuals with bulimia are of normal weight or are slightly overweight. Physical complications of bulimia nervosa are mostly related to the repeated vomiting. Stomach acid erodes the enamel of the teeth and causes sore throat. Repeated vomiting causes fluid imbalances that result in weakness and fainting and disturbances in sodium and potassium balance that can cause heart rhythm problems.

Binge-eating disorder has been proposed as a diagnosis for patients who binge but do not purge, use laxatives, or engage in other behaviors to get rid of the extra calories. As might be expected, many of these people are overweight.

The treatment of bulimia nervosa includes helping patients identify the precipitating factors of a binge, addressing their distorted body image and abnormal attitudes towards food, and teaching them healthy eating habits and coping patterns other than bingeing during periods of emotional distress.

UNDERSTANDING EATING DISORDERS

Like substance-abuse problems, eating disorders are best understood as complex, self-reinforcing *behaviors* that entrap vulnerable individuals. The challenge to understanding eating disorders in this way is that of understanding how self-starvation and the grotesque habit of bingeing and purging can possibly be self-reinforcing, that is, why patients, on some level at least, are *attracted* to these behaviors in the same way substance abusers are attracted to alcohol and drug use. It helps to first identify the vulnerabilities that are the "setup" for these behaviors.

Social and cultural factors are very important. Eating disorders are seen almost exclusively in industrialized countries where food shortage is not significant. Western culture's glorification of thinness in females is also a very important factor. One need only glance through any magazine marketed to teenagers to see the idealized feminine physique: willowy thin supermodels or buxom but toned and wiry beach beauties—often photographed and touched up in such a way as to make them look even thinner than they are in "real life." Surveys show that up to 70 percent of young women in Northern Europe and the United States feel they are overweight even when they are thin or normal in weight. Most girls simply do not have the genetic endowment needed to look like the women they constantly see depicted in magazines, on billboards, and in films and television programs. Adolescent boys feel some of the same pressures, but the emphasis is on being muscular rather than thin. This is one of the reasons why eating disorders are thought to be so much rarer in males (and perhaps why steroid abuse is almost exclusively a problem of young men).

There is also something of a class consciousness attached to thinness, exemplified by the old saying that "a woman can never be too rich or too thin." In contrast to cultures in which food is scarce and plumpness is valued, where food is plentiful, slimness and the avoidance of obesity are valued and associated with wealth. Being overweight is associated with laziness, poor self-control, and self-indulgence; thinness is associated with good health and self-discipline. Young people constantly see and hear that thin is good and fat is bad, and they incorporate these ideals into their view of what sort of body type is attractive and desirable.

While some young people are relatively unaffected by this barrage of messages about weight and appearance, those with serious self-esteem problems can take it to heart in a very serious way. I have already discussed how adolescence is a time of difficult transitions and worries about identity and "fitting in." Fears about sexual maturation crop up for younger adolescents, and older ones may equate entering adulthood with being abandoned and isolated. The adolescent fears losing control of her life in a number of important ways and may feel ineffective and helpless to influence the outcome of these developmental processes. At this point, some adolescents become preoccupied with food and weight control to distract themselves from these frightening issues.

When they restrict their food intake and experience weight loss, these young women experience a surge of competence, self-confidence, and control. Complimentary and congratulatory comments from others on successfully losing weight further reinforce weight loss as an admirable goal. Fasting and food preoccupation become a "safe place" where the girl feels in control and knows that her efforts will pay off in predictable and measurable ways. The girl with anorexia begins to take pride in her ability to adhere to stricter, narrower, and more abnormal diets and to restrict further and further. Thinness, fasting, and exercise come to be seen as virtues and eating as a vice. The adolescent becomes intoxicated by her success at losing weight and by reaching ever more ambitious weight-loss goals.

Experiments to study the psychological effects of starvation, in which healthy volunteers have gone on extremely restricted diets, have shown that constantly hungry people begin to think about food constantly, talk about food constantly, and even have dreams about food. As her food intake decreases, the girl with anorexia experiences ever stronger, and now physiologically induced, food cravings. She finds that she must work ever harder to keep the weight off. She develops increasingly irrational fears about what would happen if she were to begin to eat normally, imagining that her body would balloon to immensely obese proportions if she were to stop restricting. More fasting leads to more craving and hunger, which leads to more food preoccupation, more fear of losing control—and this leads to more fasting. A vicious circle has developed: the anorectic has become intensely fearful of eating, and fasting is the only way she knows of to deal with her anxiety. There is no escape.

Eventually, malnutrition begins to affect brain functioning. At this point, the individual becomes physically incapable of making good decisions about eating or realizing how dangerous a situation she is in. This is why, at very low weights, hospitalization is necessary to accomplish refeeding.

Individuals with bulimia follow a comparable course. They are affected by the same sociocultural factors regarding thinness and also start out worried about their weight. They often go on diets that are unreasonable and overly strict, and their initial binges are the result of impulsive and out-of-control eating to quickly alleviate their hunger pangs. Alternatively, the binge may have developed as a means of dealing with depression, loneliness, and anxiety. In either case, binge eating becomes the coping mechanism and simultaneously the cause of shame, guilt, and disgust. The bulimic starts purging to rid herself of the physical discomfort and calories that result from the binge, but this behavior (and perhaps the weight gain that results from it as well) causes more shame and guilt, precipitating more bingeing, and another vicious cycle begins.

In the treatment of eating disorders, normal eating behaviors and healthy attitudes towards food and body need to be retaught to the patient. She must also learn new ways of coping with uncomfortable feelings and address self-image and self-esteem issues. For many of these individuals, there is also an underlying mood disorder that fuels the maladaptive coping mechanisms and that requires treatment in its own right.

MOOD DISORDERS AND EATING DISORDERS

Many people with eating disorders have mood disorders as well, mostly depression. One clinical study of American high school girls with eating disorders found that more than 80 percent of them suffered from a depressive disorder, mostly major depressive disorder.[3] Another study found that dysthymic disorder was more closely associated with eating disorders.[4] But whatever the details, the pattern is very clear: the combination of an eating disorder and a mood disorder occurs too often to be explained away as simply coincidental. The cause or causes for this finding are, however, hotly debated. There is some evidence that genetic factors are at play. A study of twin girls with anorexia nervosa found evidence that genetic risk factors are very important for the development of the eating disorder and "substantially contribute to the observed co-morbidity between anorexia nervosa and major depression."[5] Perhaps it is temperamental and personality traits such as obsessiveness or a tendency to be shy and introverted that have a genetic basis, and perhaps these traits interact with social cues to set up the adolescent female for anorectic behaviors. We know that a person's degree of impulsivity has some genetic basis and that a tendency to be impulsive is frequently seen in individuals with bulimia.

The bad feelings that arise from a mood disorder may precipitate eating disorder behaviors and sustain them over time. An Italian study of patients with bulimia found that many of them had a prodrome, or preliminary phase, to their eating disorder characterized by low self-esteem, depressed mood, loss of interest and pleasure in activities, and irritability—all symptoms of depression.[6]

It is likely that the relationship between eating disorder and mood disorders is one of complex interactions that differ from one individual to another. The optimal treatment of the combination is quite clear, however: when they occur together, *both* problems require treatment. As with the combination of substance abuse and mood disorders, treating one problem does not usually make the other go away.

Several double-blind placebo-controlled studies have shown that bulimia patients can reduce the frequency of their binges when they are prescribed antidepressant medications as part of an overall treatment plan that includes psychotherapy and therapy aimed at the eating disorder behaviors.[7] Studies on antidepressant treatment of patients with anorexia nervosa at first appeared to be less impressive, but more recent studies suggest a reason to be optimistic. It seems that antidepressants have little effect when the anorectic patient is still significantly underweight, perhaps explaining the results of studies on still-malnourished hospitalized patients that have not shown antidepressants to be of much benefit. When fluoxetine (Prozac) was given to patients who had been discharged from the hospital at normal weight, however, the medication had a significantly beneficial impact on relapse rates. Perhaps biochemical abnormalities in the brains of malnourished, underweight patients prevent antidepressant medications from working properly, and only when weight has returned to normal can medication be effective.[8]

The treatment of severe eating disorders is very complex and requires a team of experts. Severely malnourished patients are best served in psychiatric hospitals that have a special eating disorders unit and a treatment team that is experienced in the therapy of such disorders. In addition to treating the abnormal eating behaviors, all the treatment options for addressing the mood disorder that almost always accompanies an eating disorder are required: a psychiatrist skilled in the prescription of antidepressants and other medications used to treat mood disorders, experienced psychotherapists, and family therapists are all necessary to treat these complex and very dangerous illnesses.

CHAPTER 13

"Cutting" and Other Self-Harming Behaviors

I have described in the last two chapters several types of self-harming behaviors that frequently complicate mood disorders: substance abuse and eating disorders. As Drs. Paul McHugh and Phillip Slavney state in their book *The Perspectives of Psychiatry*, a disorder is something people *have* whereas a behavior is something people *do*.[1] This distinction is very important when developing a treatment plan for a psychiatric problem. Treating a disorder is often easier than stopping a behavior. In this chapter, I talk about a group of behaviors often seen in people with mood disorders, behaviors in which individuals intentionally injure themselves. "Cutting" behaviors and other forms of self-mutilation, as well as the ultimate self-harming behavior, suicide, fit into this category.

SELF-MUTILATION

This account from Jill (14 years old) appeared in the *New York Times*:

> I was in the bathroom going completely crazy, just bawling my eyes out, and I think my mom was wallpapering—there was a wallpaper cutter there. I had so much anxiety, I couldn't concentrate on anything until I somehow let that out, and not being able to let it out in words, I took the razor and started cutting my leg and I got excited about seeing my blood. It felt good

to see the blood coming out, like that was my other pain leaving me too. It felt right and it felt good for me to let it out that way.[2]

Self-mutilation is deliberate, *nonsuicidal* self-injury, usually by cutting or burning the body. By definition, it is self-injury that does not involve the desire to end one's life; the self-injury is, rather, an end in itself. It is a behavior that inspires horror and disgust and seems utterly irrational. Even suicide is, in a sense, easier to understand as possibly arising out of a desire to end suffering or out of a profound hopelessness and despair. The intentional self-infliction of pain and disfigurement, on the other hand, is incomprehensible, at least at first glance. Unfortunately, self-mutilation is not rare, and it has been estimated that "cutters" and other individuals who repeatedly harm themselves number in the millions—this behavior occurs in about a thousand persons per hundred thousand population per year.[3] The prevalence of this behavior among patients being treated for psychiatric problems is much higher, approaching one in twenty.[4] Like substance abuse and eating disorders, self-inflicted injury is a complex behavior with no single "cause." Rather, it is best understood by examining the variety of factors that are involved in its development. Self-mutilation occurs in vulnerable individuals, is precipitated by emotional distress of various types, and is then sustained by additional and usually different factors.

In this section, I discuss what has been called *repetitive* or *episodic self-mutilation*. Other forms of self-harm have been described, such as the repetitive head-banging occurring in severely retarded persons and the self-mutilation in response to hallucinations or delusional ideas in individuals with psychotic illnesses. Repetitive self-mutilation, on the other hand, occurs in nonpsychotic individuals who cannot resist impulses to harm themselves physically.

Again, it's important to stress that this is not suicidal behavior, that is, individuals are not acting out of a desire to end their life. Rather, they report that the behavior gives them rapid, though short-lived relief from a variety of uncomfortable emotional states such as depression, anxiety, and anger. They describe how, while they are actually engaging in the self-harming behavior, they go into a trancelike state called *dissociation* and do not experience pain from their actions. Usually the individual feels guilty and ashamed afterwards and attempts to conceal what he or she has done. This pattern shares many behavioral elements with the eating disorders, especially bulimic behaviors, and, in fact, many patients with repetitive self-mutilation behaviors have eating disorders too.

Secondary effects of the behaviors help sustain them. As with the eating disorders, it's quite a challenge to understand how self-mutilation can make a person feel *better* in any way and what the feelings are that draw people to hurt themselves again and again. As with eating binges, episodes of self-mutilation seem to start out with a building sense of inner tension or distress that gradually increases to a point where it is unendurable. Patients report that injuring themselves provides an instant relief of this unbearable tension. They compare the relief they experience to lancing a boil, popping the lid off a pressure cooker, or bursting a balloon. The injury focuses frustration and emotional pain in the harmful act, and some patients report a sense of regaining control of their mental state by their self-injury. This sense of relief may last for hours, and the person often goes into a deep sleep afterwards.

The range of self-injuring behaviors is broad. Some individuals make only superficial skin scratches with their fingernails or pick at skin blemishes. At the other end of the continuum are those who collect razor blades, surgical gauze, and antiseptics and make careful incisions, which they then cleanse and bandage. Burning with lit cigarettes or heated metal objects is another common method of self-harm. For some people, self-mutilation seems to be a brief, time-limited behavioral syndrome, playing out over a period of weeks or months. Only a minority of persons who repeatedly injure themselves go on to develop the sort of addiction to the behavior that can go on for years. Many of these individuals have mood disorders, but we still don't know how many mood disorder patients repetitively self-injure themselves or how many self-injuring individuals have a mood disorder. As with the eating disorders, the individuals who self-mutilate appear to be predominantly female. The most important personality vulnerability factor seems to be impulsiveness. One study of women with self-mutilating behaviors found that about half of them had a history of or later developed an eating disorder and about one-fifth had a history of alcohol or drug abuse or compulsive stealing or shoplifting.[5]

The ability of the self-mutilating behavior to shock and horrify others, especially family members, is another proposed explanation for how such behaviors develop. Rendering family members (and therapists) gasping and helpless, as these behaviors do, can be a potent and dramatic way to act out anger and replace fear and depression with feelings of power and control.

Some frightening indications suggest that the number of persons with this problem is growing, and it's fairly clear that young females are especially at risk. Articles and books in the lay press that describe and discuss "cutters" have appeared with increasing frequency.[6] There is some thought that the same kinds of social factors that influence the development of eating disorders may be at work to increase the numbers of young women who are drawn, like moths to the flame, to "cutting" behaviors. In 1992, *People* magazine published excerpts from a biography of Princess Diana that revealed not only her eating disorder behaviors but repeated episodes of cutting herself as well. Film idol (and teenage heart-throb) Johnny Depp displayed scars on his forearm and told *Details* magazine in 1993 that he cut himself with a knife to mark special times in his life.[7] Just as the glorification of thinness and the societal pervasiveness of dieting lead increasing numbers of girls to attempt to lose weight and trap a few of them into eating disorder behaviors, the glamorizing and romanticizing of self-injury in the famous may be leading more and more girls to try "cutting." The increasing prevalence and acceptance of such "body modification" behaviors as tattooing, piercing, and scarification (producing tissue injury in order to develop decorative scars) among young people may also be a factor, reducing the barriers to trying "cutting" by making painful and visible assaults on the body more acceptable.

The treatment of self-mutilation resembles that of eating disorders in that the individual must be persuaded to give up a behavior that, however perverse, is powerfully addictive. Treating underlying depression is, of course, always necessary. Therapy to identify other sources of uncomfortable emotional states and to help the individual learn alternative ways of coping with them is extremely important. Treating repetitive self-mutilation is complex and requires intensive, long-term multidisciplinary therapy, preferably by specialists in the treatment of these problems.

A promising technique for treating patients who engage in repetitive self-mutilation is a form of cognitive therapy called *dialectical-behavioral therapy* (DBT). Originated by Dr. Marsha Linehan at the University of Washington in Seattle, DBT was developed to treat individuals with repetitive self-harming behaviors of all types, including persons who make repeated suicide attempts.[8] It focuses on helping the patient identify and interrupt the thinking and emotional processes that lead up to an episode of self-mutilation and consists of weekly individual psychotherapy and group therapy sessions. There is a strong emphasis on learning how to tolerate distressing emotional states, on learning to better regulate emotions, and especially on changing behavior patterns to eliminate self-harm. For adolescents who have repetitive problems with self-mutilation, seeking out a therapist who is trained and experienced in DBT is probably well worth the effort.

In the introduction to an issue of a psychiatric research periodical devoted to the topic of self-mutilation, the scientific editor, a well-known psychiatrist, stated, "The typical clinician treating a patient who self-mutilates is often left feeling a combination of helpless, horrified, guilty, furious, betrayed, disgusted and sad."[9] As in treating other destructive but addictive behaviors, the intense and specialized treatment is often difficult and time-consuming; recovery can be frustratingly slow. Fortunately, more and more research on the causes and correlates of this syndrome is being done, and the number of therapists who are skilled in its treatment is increasing.

ADOLESCENT SUICIDE

In the chapters in this part of the book, I have been discussing complex behaviors that often complicate mood disorders but that are shaped and precipitated by many factors and influences—behaviors that do not have any simple "cause." Suicidal behavior also falls into this category.

I discuss the danger signals of an impending suicide and talk about suicide prevention later in this book (chapter 16). Here I want to discuss the adolescent suicide a bit more abstractly and address some misconceptions about suicide in this age group.

The rates of suicide among adolescents rose steadily in the United States during the second half of the twentieth century. In 1956, the completed suicide rate among 15- to 19-year-olds was just over 2 per 100,000 individuals per year, a number that turned out to be the lowest of the century. By the mid-1980s, this number had increased nearly fivefold, to about 11 per 100,000 per year. Most strikingly, boys almost entirely accounted for this dramatic increase in the number of adolescent suicides, with the suicide rate for males in this age range approaching 20 per 100,000 per year in 1988. In the last decade of the century, there were some encouraging suggestions that this rate had started dropping slightly. During this entire, almost fifty-year period, the suicide rate for adults aged 30 to 60 remained fairly constant at 15 or 16 per 100,000 persons per year.[10]

The number of adolescents who make *suicide attempts* is far larger than the number who actually kill themselves. For every adolescent who commits suicide, more than a hundred others have made an attempt. Most of these attempts do not result in any injuries and many are medically inconsequential, such as taking a handful of aspirin tablets or making superficial scratches on the wrists. Studies have indicated that only about 2 to 3 percent of adolescents who have made a suicide attempt seek medical treatment. Studies also show that twice as many adolescent girls make a suicide attempt as boys, but more than five times more boys than girls actually kill themselves. It has been suggested that those who *attempt* suicide and those who succeed in killing themselves are two different though, of course, overlapping groups. But a review of the research studies on individuals who make suicide attempts and on those who die from completed suicide reveals that, aside from the differences in sex ratio, the characteristics of the two groups don't appear so terribly different clinically. Also, most adolescents who actually kill themselves have previously made a suicide attempt. It appears that both groups usually suffer from psychiatric problems, most especially mood disorders.

For many years, mental health experts held on to what might be called the "Romeo and Juliet" theory of adolescent suicide, the idea that adolescence is a time of stress and that any individual exposed to an intolerable amount of psychological stress is at risk for suicide. The theory was a natural outgrowth of the early *Sturm und Drang* ideas about adolescence that I discussed in chapter 2: that all adolescents are volatile, impulsive, and raging with emotions, and those who attempt suicide are, like Romeo and Juliet, simply more volatile and impulsive and under greater environmental stress. This is clearly not the case. The vast majority of adolescent suicide victims suffer from a mood disorder. Environmental stressors seem to play some role in the behavior, but the underlying psychiatric illness appears to be the most important factor. For this reason, suicide prevention programs aimed at adolescents are beginning to shift away from "stress management" models to programs that educate adolescents and their families on how to recognize mood disorder symptoms and on the importance of treatment.

One model for understanding and preventing adolescent suicide that is increasingly accepted in psychiatry is that developed by David Shaffer and his colleagues at Columbia University in New York. This multifactorial model proposes that suicidal thinking originates in an adolescent because of an underlying psychiatric disorder, but it smolders under the surface until more active consideration of suicide is precipitated by some stressful event; at that point, actual suicidal behavior is either facilitated or inhibited by a combination of mostly external factors (see figure 13-1).

Numerous studies have found that almost all adolescents who commit suicide suffer from depression, forming the basis for the proposed first step

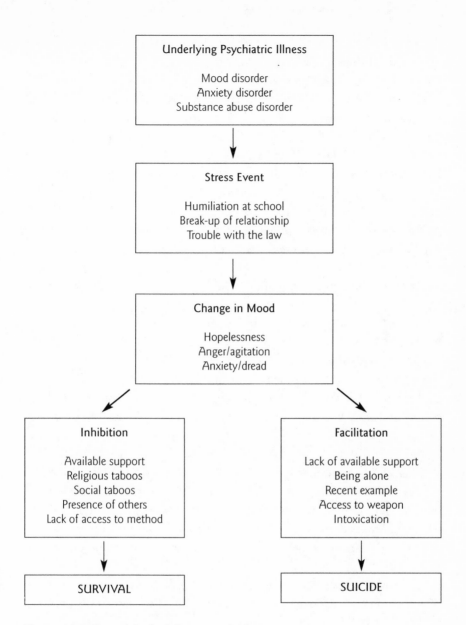

Figure 13-1 A model of adolescent suicide
Source: Described in David Shaffer and Leslie Craft, "Methods of Adolescent Suicide Prevention," *Journal of Clinical Psychiatry* 60, suppl. 2 (1999): 70–74.

of this model: development of an underlying psychiatric disorder. Studies of adolescent suicides indicate that the most common underlying disorders are mood disorders. In boys, a combination of a mood disorder and a substance-abuse problem is especially dangerous. In a study of 120 adolescent suicide victims, in which the investigators reviewed medical records and interviewed parents, friends, and teachers to make a psychiatric diagnosis of the victims, the factors that best predicted suicide were the diagnoses of a mood disorder and a substance-abuse disorder and a previous history of a suicide attempt.[11] Often, the victims had shown symptoms of these disorders for several years before their suicide.

The suicide attempt is precipitated in these vulnerable individuals by what Shaffer calls a *stress event*, an event such as being in trouble with the police or at school, for example, or the breakup of a relationship or simply a recent distressing or humiliating experience. Often the stress event can be understood in relation to the underlying disorder: the stress event leads to an acute emotional crisis with the development of extreme anxiety, dread, and hopelessness; a sense of inner tension and agitation builds, and the adolescent feels compelled to "do something."

At this point, external factors serve either to facilitate or to inhibit suicidal behavior. A strong religious belief about the sinfulness of suicide would be an inhibitory factor, whereas living in a culture where suicide is seen as an acceptable solution to problems (as was formerly the case in Japan) would be facilitating. The availability of a supportive, trusted influence such as a family member, a close friend, or a therapist to help soothe and decompress the situation would be an inhibiting factor. Studies suggest that feelings of connectedness to family are protective against suicide. Being or feeling isolated and unable to reach out for comfort or support, on the other hand, appears to be a facilitator. This factor has been cited as important in understanding the much higher rate of suicidal behavior among adolescents who experience questions and conflicts over same-sex romantic attraction and who feel unable to discuss this issue with family, friends, or the other usual sources of support.[12]

Another facilitating factor is the recent suicide of someone known to the adolescent or even someone simply living in the same community, serving as a model for suicidal behavior. The issue of *suicide contagion* has received attention: the observation that adolescent suicides often occur in clusters and that the suicide of one adolescent can lead to a series of others. In February 1990, a physician notified the Centers for Disease Control (CDC), the federal agency that investigates epidemics and the spread of illnesses, that two adolescent boys had committed suicide in Santa Fe County, New Mexico, within four days of each other. The New Mexico Department of Health investigated and found that the number of persons under the age of 20 who had been evaluated for a suicide attempt or suicidal thinking had *tripled* that month, a finding interpreted as strongly suggesting that one suicide can lead others to make an attempt. The study also found that the rate of suicide attempts had been consistently lower during June, July, and August for the preceding three years, giving support to the idea that school problems can be a precipitating factor for suicidal behavior.[13] Other clusters have been identified as well in other parts of the country.

Media coverage of an adolescent suicide that seeks to comfort a community may have the unwanted effect of promoting the clustering of suicides. Portrayals of a poignant family and community tragedy with emotional descriptions of grieving friends and family, and of moving eulogies given at well-attended funerals, have the effect of presenting suicide in a positive way and making it more acceptable. In 1994, the CDC issued media guidelines for reporting on suicide and listed several aspects of media coverage that may promote suicide contagion, including presenting simplistic explanations for suicide or presenting suicide as an understandable way of coping with personal problems ("John had recently broken up with his girlfriend"). Focusing on the victim's accomplishments and positive characteristics is also discouraged, as it may make suicide more attractive to vulnerable adolescents who feel that those around them do not appreciate them.

Other suicide facilitators include opportunity and access factors, such as being alone at home and the availability of a highly lethal suicide method, such as access to a gun. Most adolescents who kill themselves use a gun, and it is quite clear that the presence of a firearm in the home greatly increases the risk of suicide. One study showed that the presence of *any* firearm increased adolescent suicide risk, and whether the weapon was a handgun or a long gun, kept loaded or unloaded, locked up or not, made no difference.[14]

Perhaps the ultimate facilitating factor is intoxication of some type. Not only does a substance-abuse diagnosis greatly increase the risk of suicide, but most persons who kill themselves have alcohol in their bloodstream when they do so. It has been suggested that the increase in the number of adolescent suicides is due to the increasing numbers of teenagers who have access to alcohol and illegal drugs.

Public health efforts at suicide prevention are increasingly focusing on the start of the process that leads to suicide: identifying the psychiatric disorder and getting the adolescent into treatment. Although "hot lines" and crisis services have been popular efforts, there is little research evidence to suggest they have much impact on suicide rates in a community. Nor do efforts to educate high school students and parents about the self-identification of depression and referral for treatment show any clear impact. Actually screening students for symptoms of depression and suicidal thinking and making further evaluation and treatment available to students who screen positive may be the most effective means of reducing suicide rates in the community. A 1999 study evaluated the effectiveness of a computer questionnaire that screened for symptoms of depression and suicidal thinking in identifying at-risk adolescents, who were then referred for more thorough evaluation. The study found that almost a third of the students identified as suffering from major depression were receiving no treatment.[15]

Recent data indicate that the adolescent suicide rate peaked in the late 1980s and may be starting to drop. This coincided with the introduction of more effective SSRI antidepressant medications, and some have suggested that improved treatment of serious depression in adolescents may be an important factor in this welcome trend. However, many factors are at work, and much research into the causes and solutions of this problem remains to be done before the startling epidemic of adolescent suicide of the last fifty years or so can be said to be under control.

CHAPTER 14

The Genetics of Mood Disorders

As has long been recognized, mood disorders cluster within families. In his landmark textbook of psychiatry, Dr. Emil Kraepelin, who more or less invented the modern concept of mood disorders, wrote of one family in which "of the ten children of the same parents who were both probably manic-depressive by predisposition, no fewer than seven fell ill the same way; of the five descendants of the second generation, four have already fallen ill."[1]

For many years, research on the genetics of mood disorders was hampered by foggy diagnostic criteria and a lack of laboratory methods to identify genes. But this is changing. Not only have psychiatrists become more skilled in the diagnosis of mood disorders, but the biochemical methods available to locate and identify genes on the human chromosomes have become tremendously more sophisticated. These developments will, sooner or later, lead to a better understanding of the genetic mechanisms of mood disorders, which will in turn lead to better diagnosis and treatment of these illnesses.

GENES, CHROMOSOMES, AND DNA

A brief discussion of the principles of genetics, the scientific study of the inheritance of biological attributes, is necessary before turning to a discussion of the heredity of mood disorders.

The patterns and rules of inheritance in living things were first described by Gregor Mendel, an Austrian monk who, over many years, performed elegantly planned and executed experiments with plants, mostly garden peas, in his monastery garden. Prior to Mendel's work in the latter half of the nineteenth century, it was thought that the traits of one parent were simply blended with those of the other parent in their offspring, who thus had traits that were intermediate between those of the two parents. Mendel discovered that this was not always or even usually true. He found, for example, that crossing a pea plant that produced tall plants with a pea plant that produced short ones (which he did by transferring pollen from one plant to the other) did not give rise to seeds that produced medium plants—that is, an intermediate form. Instead, Mendel discovered that *all* the seeds formed from this cross gave rise to tall plants. When he then crossed the offspring plants and planted the next generation of seed, exactly *three-quarters* of them produced tall plants and *one-quarter* produced short plants. There were no intermediate forms and no blending of traits. The offspring received either a "tall" inheritance or a "short" one—there were no "in-betweens." Mendel concluded that each parent contributed something that determined plant size, and these "somethings" were distributed to the next generation and determined plant size in that generation. These "somethings" are now called *genes*, the units of inheritance.

We now understand that genes are sets of instructions for building proteins. All plants and animals are constructed (in part) and operate by means of proteins. Myosin (muscle protein), hemoglobin (the oxygen-carrying protein of red blood cells), and collagen (the structural protein of skin and cartilage) are just a few examples. Even the nonprotein structural materials of the body, such as the calcium salts in our bones, depend on proteins. Proteins called enzymes direct the manufacture of bone from calcium salts by expediting certain chemical reactions. Many hormones are proteins (insulin, for example) and those that are not (such as testosterone and cortisol) are manufactured by protein enzymes. I've already mentioned some members of the protein family that are of enormous interest to those studying mood disorders: G proteins and the receptors for neurotransmitters. All proteins are built according to specifications contained in genes.

For many years, it was believed that genes were proteins also, that is, that genetic information was somehow encoded in protein molecules. But by the mid-1940s, experiments with bacteria had proven that a far simpler family of biochemical compounds, called *nucleic acids*, contained the genetic information. In 1953, James Watson and Francis Crick published a paper in the British scientific journal *Nature* describing the structure of the most important of these compounds, deoxyribonucleic acid (DNA). With this discovery, the modern age of genetics had begun.

DNA molecules are long spiral chains, their "links" consisting of four simpler compounds called nucleotides. The four types of DNA nucleotides, containing adenine, cytosine, guanine, and thymine (usually abbreviated as A, C, G, and T), are the elements of an elegantly simple code used to write out instructions for the manufacture of proteins. Just as you can write out a Morse code version of *Hamlet* using only dots and dashes, you can write out instructions for building hemoglobin, myosin, collagen, or any other protein using A's, C's, G's and T's. That's what DNA does. You can think of the physical structure of a gene as the section of a DNA molecule that codes for one protein.

When the DNA molecule is doing its work in the cell, it is unraveled and stretched out and surrounded by a whole retinue of ultramicroscopic attendants busily reading the coded instructions and making proteins. When it's time for the cell to divide, another set of attendants carefully coil the DNA molecule into a compact cylinder and surround it with protective proteins to form the threadlike structures you probably looked at under the microscope in high school biology: the chromosomes.

GENETIC DISEASES

Sometimes the pathways from a certain gene to a certain protein to a certain trait or disease are easy to follow (although, in medicine, as we'll see, the understanding of these paths has usually been approached from the other direction: disease to protein to gene). Sickle-cell anemia is one disease for which the pathway from gene to disease is easy to follow. If you looked at the blood of a person with sickle-cell anemia under the microscope, instead of seeing the normal saucer-shaped red blood cells, you'd see abnormal crescent-shaped (sickle-shaped) cells. When scientists had the biochemical methods to look at the components of blood cells, they discovered that people with sickle-cell anemia had an abnormally shaped hemoglobin molecule, which tended to form abnormal chains within the cell, stretching the normally disk-shaped cells into the characteristic sickle shape seen under the microscope.

Because hemoglobin is easily purified, it was one of the first proteins whose structure was completely described (a feat that earned Cambridge

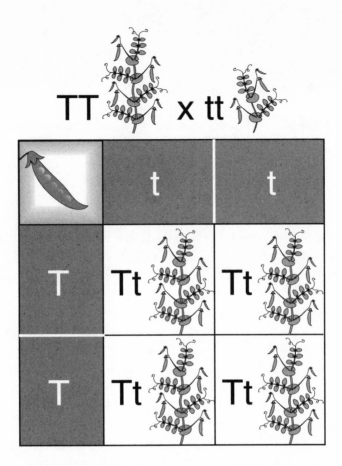

TT × tt

Figure 14-1 *Above*: Mendel's cross between a tall (*TT*) and a short (*tt*) pea plant. Each offspring (seed) receives two tallness genes, one from each parent plant. The seeds from this cross grew all tall plants because all received the *tall* gene (*T*), which dominates over the *short* gene (*t*). *At right*: When the next generation of plants is crossed, one-fourth of them receive no *tall* gene (*T*) and therefore grow short plants.

University biochemist Max Ferdinand Perutz the Nobel Prize in 1962). Sickle-cell hemoglobin (hemoglobin S) was found to differ from normal hemoglobin by only a few atoms, the equivalent of a single substitution of one nucleotide for another in the gene of the DNA molecule. Because of a number of biochemical factors that made the hemoglobin gene especially accessible and easy to work with, scientists could pinpoint its location early on in the search for genes that caused human diseases. We now know that

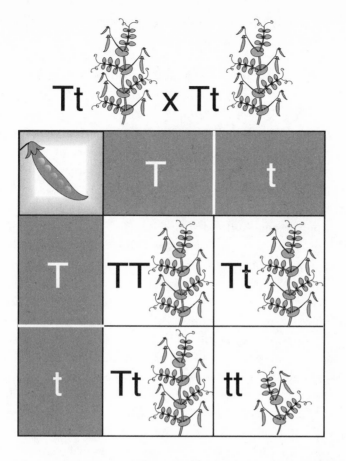

at one particular spot on the DNA molecule of persons who have sickle-cell anemia, there is an A instead of a T in the set of instructions. An abnormal hemoglobin molecule results from the reading of these incorrect instructions. The abnormal hemoglobin causes the abnormally shaped red blood cells, which block blood vessels and result in the symptoms of the disease. The pathway from abnormal gene to abnormal protein to abnormal cells to symptoms was completely described.

Genes have been identified and located for several other human diseases whose inheritance pattern indicates that they are single-gene illnesses. In some cases, this has been possible even though the identity or function of the protein the abnormal gene codes for is unknown. Huntington's disease (or Huntington's chorea), the degenerative brain disease that afflicted folk-singer Woody Guthrie and his family, is one example.

Scientists searching for "disease genes" now often use *linkage studies* to locate and identify genes. These studies take advantage of the fact that genes located close to one another on the same chromosome tend to stay together when the chromosomes undergo the process that apportions them into egg or sperm cells. In linkage studies, geneticists take advantage of gene maps that show the location of marker genes. First, DNA tests are performed on a blood sample of persons with the condition being investigated as well as on unaffected family members. Scientists then perform sophisticated mathematical analyses of the presence or absence of marker genes in affected and unaffected subjects to find an association between the condition and marker genes. If an association is found, the known location of the markers pinpoints the location of the gene for the condition. This method has been highly successful in locating the genes for several other single-gene diseases, including cystic fibrosis and Duchenne muscular dystrophy.

Studies have indicated that depressive disorders and bipolar mood disorders are probably related genetically at least some of the time. Serious depression is two to ten times more likely to occur among relatives of persons with bipolar disorder than in families of persons who don't have the illness. When one examines the family tree of persons with major depressive disorder, the data are not quite as clear; more persons with bipolar disorder than would be expected are found in some studies but not in others. This has been interpreted as indicating that when major depressive disorder shows up in families with bipolar disorder, the depressive illness is genetically similar to bipolar disorder, but that depressive illness in the absence of bipolar disorder in the family has more varied causes and may or may not share the same genes as bipolar disorder.

When several genes might be involved in an illness, the problem of gene identification becomes tremendously more complicated. And if the illness takes several forms or is difficult to diagnose, the task becomes monumental. Unfortunately, all of this applies to mood disorders. Most scientists looking for genetic causes of mood disorders agree that these are not one-gene illnesses like sickle-cell anemia or Huntington's disease. Mood disorders are caused, in all probability, by several different genes, perhaps as many as a dozen or so. The illnesses take many different forms and are sometimes difficult to diagnose.

In the late 1980s, several reports appeared that purported to link a mood disorder, specifically bipolar disorder, to specific regions of chromosomes. The most significant report was of an Amish family that seemed to carry a gene for bipolar disorder on one end of chromosome 11 (human cells have twenty-two pairs of chromosomes, numbered 1 through 22, and a pair of sex chromosomes). In this study, the researchers thought they had overcome at least one of the usual hurdles to finding a "bipolar gene." This particular family pedigree seemed to indicate Mendelian, that is, single-gene, inheritance at work. Even if there were several possible genes that could cause bipolar disorder, this particular family seemed to pass on the disorder through only one gene. Mathematical analysis of previously identified DNA markers pointed to chromosome 11, and the statistical significance of the findings appeared solid. Zeroing in on a mood disorder gene seemed within reach.

Within just months, however, these results were called into question when another team of scientists took another look at the mathematical analysis. But it was the issue of diagnosis that ultimately scuttled this ambitious study. Several of the individuals who had been classified as unaffected when the data were originally collected developed symptoms of bipolar disorder later on. When the new numbers were "crunched," the results fell apart completely.[2]

Linkage studies have pointed to a number of different locations on different chromosomes as possible sites for "mood disorder genes," but results are still preliminary and sometimes, as with the Amish study, repeat testing has cast doubt on the conclusions (although work on chromosome 18 looks very encouraging).[3]

Looking for genes involved in major depressive disorder has been even more difficult, because this disorder can be even more difficult to diagnose. Studies of *childhood-onset* major depressive disorder, however, have demonstrated that this form of the illness is especially likely to run in families, suggesting that studies of the childhood-onset illness will prove the most useful for studying genes for major depression.

People who develop mood disorder symptoms most likely have inherited *several* genes that predispose them to these illnesses. There is even some thought that these are relatively common genes that many people carry without ever developing a mood disorder. Perhaps a certain number of genetic "hits" are necessary to make a person vulnerable to developing mood disorder symptoms, and perhaps certain environmental conditions are needed as well. These factors make the search for mood disorder genes all the more daunting.

WHAT WE KNOW

Until we identify specific genes and discover what proteins these genes code for, we can talk about the inheritance of mood disorders in only a very general way. What we can say is that the children of persons with mood disorders have an increased risk of developing a mood disorder. Assigning a number to that risk is very difficult, owing to some of the same problems that have made the search for mood disorder genes so difficult, especially problems of diagnosis. But the risk appears to be several times that for the general population, on the order of 10 percent for those with a family history of the disease. The risks in bipolar disorder can be quantified more precisely. The chance of developing bipolar disorder for a child who has a parent with bipolar disorder also appears to be several times that for the general population, again on the order of 10 percent. However, children of persons with bipolar disorder are also at a higher risk for unipolar (depression only) illness, and when you add this risk in, the percentages go up into the high twenties. This means that the children of persons with bipolar disorder have about a one in four chance of developing some kind of mood disorder and about a one in ten chance of developing bipolar disorder.[4]

Persons with mood disorders need to be alert to signs and symptoms of mood disorders in their children and get them into treatment if these signs appear. Although we may be uncertain about the details of the inheritance of these illnesses, we are not at all uncertain about the importance of early diagnosis and treatment.

THE SEARCH CONTINUES

Several factors make scientists optimistic about eventually discovering genes for mood disorders. In 1999, scientists of the Human Genome Project and Celera Genomics announced the "first draft" of the full sequence of human chromosomal DNA. Specifically, the pattern of A's, C's, G's, and T's in human DNA had been worked out. As important as this accomplishment is, all human genes and their locations have *not* yet been determined.

But the number of identified genetic markers used in the linkage studies that *will* determine gene locations continues to rise. These markers, like signposts along the length of the chromosome, designate particular locations in the DNA molecule: the more genetic signposts there are, the easier it will be to find a particular gene. More precise diagnoses will also help, as will the study of larger family pedigrees and development of techno-logical advances—both biochemical methods and more powerful com-puters and software to do the mathematical analyses.

Even when genes are identified and tests developed that can look for these genes in individuals, predictions about who will develop symptoms will probably still be imprecise. This is because several genes are likely in-volved and also because genetics is unlikely to be the whole story. Envi-ronmental factors are probably operating to determine who will and will not be affected: psychological and perhaps physical stresses and traumas may be very important. Some evidence suggests that viruses play a role in the development of some psychiatric disorders. So even when a gene or genes are identified and can be tested for, finding that a person has a mood disorder gene will probably mean that she has a much higher chance of de-veloping symptoms than someone who does not have the gene, but devel-oping them is not a certainty—the risk is not 100 percent. This will raise many difficult questions about who should and should not be tested and who is entitled to know the test results (siblings? spouse? employers? in-surance companies?).[5]

But finding the genes responsible for mood disorders may lead to new treatment approaches that will benefit everyone with these illnesses. Gene identification, and identification of the function of these genes or their gene products, will undoubtedly shed light on the biochemical basis of mood disorders. It may then be possible to design medications or other treatments based on knowledge about the causes of symptoms at the cellular or bio-chemical level—rather than stumbling upon treatments by accident as has been the case so far. Genetics research is one of the most challenging but also the most promising areas of investigation of mood disorders and holds the promise of truly revolutionizing the treatment of these illnesses.

Keep in mind that depression and other mood disorders of adolescence are not "cured" by any of the treatments discussed in part II of this book. We are getting better and better at treating these problems, but talk of cures is still years, perhaps even decades, in the future. In the meantime, however, there are many things that can be done to promote good mental health. Millions of individuals have been diagnosed with mood disorders and are living happy, healthy, and productive lives. Unfortunately, many are not. These chapters are intended to help you and your adolescent maximize the chances of staying in the first category and out of the second.

But if you're looking for a simple list of dos and don'ts, I'm afraid you will be disappointed. Instead, in chapter 15 I've tried to lay out some general principles that underlie the sorts of advice and recommendations usually given to patients in the doctor's office or clinic. I hope that after reading this chapter, you'll have a better understanding of why some of the dos and don'ts that you hear from the doctor and therapist are so important.

Adolescent depression doesn't just affect the teenager. Inevitably, family members are affected in countless ways, both directly and indirectly, and chapter 16 addresses this aspect of the illness. I'll go over what family members can do—and just as important, what family members cannot and should not try to do—to help their loved one who has a mood disorder.

In chapter 17, I've collected together some principles for dealing with emergencies and highlighted the types of emergency situations that, in my experience, patients and their families often fail to prepare for. It's so tempting to put off thinking about and planning for things that we hope won't happen; I emphasize in this chapter how important it is not to give in to this temptation and how easy it is to be prepared for emergencies.

Finally, I provide a short chapter that looks into the future and explores some of the exciting possibilities that may help us to better understand mood disorders. With this knowledge, it should be possible to improve the diagnosis and treatment of these illnesses, and perhaps one day we might be able to cure them.

CHAPTER 15

Strategies for Successful Treatment

This chapter presents some principles of good treatment for mood disorders in adolescents. In depression and bipolar disorder, perhaps as in no other kind of medical problem, treatment must be carefully tailored to each patient's needs. In part III of this book, I indicated how complex treatment can be when a person has complicating problems such as substance abuse or an eating disorder along with a depressive disorder. But even when these complications are not in the picture, the best treatment approach to adolescent depression is often a matter of much dispute. Experts frequently disagree on what should be considered standard treatments for these illnesses, which often makes treating patients more of an art than a science.

The prescription of medications for the treatment of adolescents with mood disorders is frequently "off-label" (see chapter 5), and new medications are being touted all the time as useful for treating mood disorders (though often on the basis of a few case reports). How should parents make decisions about medication, about choosing a therapist, about hospitalizing their child? How can parents know whether their child is receiving the best possible treatment?

Because these illnesses are so complex and poorly understood, I cannot say which medication should always be tried first or tell you at what point another pharmaceutical or an additional one should be tried. But I can lay out some principles that underlie successful treatment and that will usually, though perhaps only slowly, put your youngster on the road to recovery.

DIAGNOSIS, DIAGNOSIS, DIAGNOSIS

You've probably heard the old saw that the three most important factors in the real estate business are location, location, location. A similar saying would be well heeded by all mental health professionals: the three most important factors in the development of a treatment plan in medicine are diagnosis, diagnosis, diagnosis.

Occasionally, I speak to a parent who is interested in getting a consultation about her adolescent's problems and who tells me something like, "Our son has been diagnosed with major depressive disorder, ADHD, obsessive-compulsive disorder, generalized anxiety, separation anxiety, and a learning disorder, and his therapist is wondering if he's not developing a personality disorder, too. We want to be sure he's getting the proper treatment for all his diagnoses so that doesn't happen." Not infrequently, the adolescent is on a different medication for *each* of his "diagnoses" and is experiencing so many side effects that any kind of normal functioning is impossible.

This problem with accumulating diagnoses in psychiatry seems to me to be a direct result of the "checklist" method of the DSM, which lists different symptoms of various disorders and asks for several from this column and a few from that one to meet diagnostic criteria. It's very easy to go through these various diagnostic checklists and, before you know it, a whole collection of "diagnoses" is on the patient's chart. But this is not what the diagnostic process is all about. Rather, the job of the diagnostician is to put together *all* the information about symptoms, family history, medical history, and the findings on examining the patient in order to formulate a coherent diagnostic impression that pulls together the entire story—in *one* diagnosis if possible.

The overlap of the symptoms of bipolar disorder and ADHD is a good example of how this kind of diagnostic confusion can develop. Some of the symptoms of ADHD, such as impulsivity, impatience, disorganized thinking, and poor concentration, are, of course, also seen in adolescents with bipolar disorder. These are distressing symptoms that deserve attention, but more importantly, they deserve the right kind of attention. If they are an expression of the mood changes of bipolar disorder, then medication for ADHD won't help. (In fact, the medications used to treat ADHD, stimulants and antidepressants, can make things worse.) Adolescents with depression are especially vulnerable to irritable mood states that lead to behavioral problems that might suggest an additional diagnosis of conduct disorder or oppositional defiant disorder. I want to persuade you that giving these youngsters additional *diagnoses* often doesn't clarify their situation; it just confuses the picture.

When I see a patient who seems to have too many diagnoses, I wonder about how much information-gathering and critical thinking went into the diagnostic process. The same applies when there seem to be too many medications. Does the patient really have several different disorders that need treatment with different medications—an antidepressant for depression, a tranquilizer for anxiety, a mood stabilizer for "mood swings," and so on? Or have too many medications accumulated to treat various manifestations of one disorder?

Making a diagnosis is the process of attempting to identify the one process that can explain all the patient's symptoms. There is a scientific principle called "Occam's razor," named after the medieval theologian-philosopher who developed it, William of Occam (or Ockham). This principle states that the simplest explanation for a phenomenon is always preferable to a more complex one and is more likely to be correct. Obviously, a patient may have two or three or four different disorders that require different treatment approaches. But if all the symptoms can be understood as expressions of *one* disorder, treating that one will likely alleviate all the symptoms. Even when there are clearly several problems, formulating the relationship between them often makes the treatment plan priorities clear. For example, an adolescent may have a depressive disorder that is "fueling" eating disorder behaviors and precipitating alcohol abuse. These three problems all need attention, but unless the depression that is driving the behavioral problems is aggressively treated, treatment aimed solely at behavioral problems will not be very effective. I have seen many young people go through extensive (and expensive) substance-abuse rehabilitation programs only to relapse as soon as they leave the program, because a mood disorder underlying the substance-abuse problem was never identified and properly treated.

Another diagnostic pitfall is putting too much emphasis on psychological testing and rating scales. I occasionally see parents who have been told their child has a particular psychiatric diagnosis solely on the basis of psychological testing (meaning "paper-and-pencil" testing) or even of a score on some rating scale administered by someone. Frequently parents think this is the definitive diagnostic procedure.

Sometimes parents insist that psychological testing be administered to their child as part of the assessment. Rating scales and psychological testing are helpful tools for the diagnostic process, but they are not sufficient in themselves to make a psychiatric diagnosis and are rarely the final answer to the diagnostic process. Many people think that a psychological test is like an x-ray: by means of trick questions and other mysterious methods, a psychological test will reveal what's "really" there, just as an x-ray can reveal a break in a bone that is otherwise undetectable. This is nonsense. Most psychological tests simply compare the way an individual answers standardized test questions with the way groups of others have answered the same questions, then assume that the individual being tested resembles the group whose answer patterns are closest to his answers. Psychological tests are useful for helping to identify personality styles quickly, but they don't do a very good job of making diagnoses of psychiatric disorders. A depression rating scale might show that someone is depressed, and might even be able to say whether he is mildly or severely depressed, but it won't do a very good job of telling whether he is suffering from major depressive disorder, bipolar depression, dysthymic disorder, or more minor temporary depression. And when a person is depressed, psychological tests aren't even very good at what they usually do best—revealing personality style—as the depression will alter the profile of answers. If the individual being tested isn't very honest in completing questions, the results will be practically meaningless.

This is not to say that psychological testing is never useful. It is very accurate and precise in grading people on the mental abilities that we call intelligence. The same goes for tests of memory, some types of problem-solving abilities, and other types of mental functioning. Paper-and-pencil tests are also helpful in screening large groups of people for the possibility that they might have some psychiatric disorder, identifying those who need a more in-depth evaluation for a particular problem. Various rating scales are useful in assessing changes in the severity of a disorder's symptoms over time. An individual who is suffering from depression might fill out a depression rating scale at each visit to the doctor or therapist, who can then make a more accurate assessment of progress, or lack of it, by following how the scores change over time.

The decision to give an adolescent an antidepressant cannot be made on the basis of a depression questionnaire. The diagnosis of attention-deficit/hyperactivity disorder cannot be made on the basis of a score on a screening test for ADHD. A battery of psychological tests is rarely necessary for the accurate diagnosis of mood disorders; a thorough psychiatric assessment is sufficient (and, as I will make clear in the next section, necessary). Like any other laboratory test, a psychological test can answer a specific question that comes up during a psychiatric assessment (How intelligent is this person? How introverted is this person compared with most people?). But putting an individual through a battery of tests to "see what shows up" is not good practice.

One last warning about the diagnostic process. In a very popular book for parents about mood disorders in young people, I read something to the effect that parents should be wary of a doctor who "takes too long to make a diagnosis." I am going to tell you the very opposite: beware of a doctor or therapist who seems too eager to make a diagnosis, especially multiple diagnoses, too quickly. Adolescent mood disorders are often complex, subtle, and difficult to diagnose, especially if the adolescent has come to treatment reluctantly or has trouble describing how she feels. If there are complicating factors like substance abuse or behavioral problems, it may take several visits over a period of weeks or even months to get the best sense of how the various problems relate to each other and what the best treatment approach should be.

CHOOSING THE TREATMENT TEAM

I hope I have convinced you by now that adolescent-onset depressive disorders are serious illnesses that require serious treatment by specialists. The foregoing section should make it clear that the diagnostic process is vitally important in starting treatment on the right track. For that reason, a full evaluation by a psychiatrist should be part of the treatment process as early as possible. There are places for many different types of professionals in the treatment of depression, but the point of entry needs to be with an individual who has the most training and experience in the treatment of psychiatric illnesses: a psychiatrist.

Psychiatrists have attended medical school, where they have learned about the structure and biological functioning of the human body (anatomy and physiology), the biological chemistry of the body and the principles of treatment with medication (pharmacology and therapeutics), the methods for examining bodily and mental functioning by physical examination, mental status examination, laboratory tests, and medical imaging (x-rays, MRI scans [magnetic resonance imaging], and other methods), as well as the principles of treating medical and surgical diseases. After medical school, psychiatrists train in the specialty of psychiatry for four years, applying what they have learned in medical school about diagnosis and treatment of disease to the evaluation and treatment of psychiatric problems of all types. They also learn a set of therapeutic skills that are somewhat different from those of their colleagues in other medical specialties: the principles of psychotherapy. By studying the works of behavioral scientists — Freud, Erikson, and others — psychiatrists learn about the theories of psychology, and by counseling and doing therapy with patients, they learn the practice of psychotherapy. Some individuals take additional training in the diagnosis and treatment of psychiatric problems in children and adolescents, usually a two-year program (called a *fellowship*) in child and adolescent psychiatry. At the conclusion of their training, most psychiatrists apply for certification by the American Board of Psychiatry and Neurology. They undergo a day of written tests and a day of oral examinations by experienced psychiatrists, who personally observe the applicant examine patients and then question him or her about diagnosis and treatment. Applicants who pass these rigorous examinations are said to be "board certified." A psychiatrist may also apply for a specialty certificate in child and adolescent psychiatry, a certification that requires additional testing.

A *psychotherapist* is anyone who does counseling and psychotherapy. Thus a psychotherapist may have a variety of professional education and training experiences. A *psychologist* has a university degree in the science of human behavior: psychology. The field of psychology covers the whole range of mental life and functioning: language development, how visual images are represented in the brain, the neural basis of learning, crowd behaviors, and the accurate measurement of intelligence — these are only a few of the areas within this immense and fascinating field. Psychologists may focus on understanding normal human — or animal — behaviors through research (experimental psychology) or on the dynamics of groups of individuals (organizational psychology) or on the treatment of psychological problems (clinical psychology). *Clinical psychology* is the subspecialty of the field involved in the treatment of emotional problems. A clinical psychologist usually has a four-year college or university degree plus several more years of education towards a master's degree or a Ph.D. (doctorate) degree. Clinical psychologists have focused on theories of human behavior as they relate to the development of psychological problems, have learned various methods of psychological assessment (such as giving and scoring intelligence tests, personality assessments, and other tests of mental functioning), and have learned about psychological disorders and psychological treatments: counseling and psychotherapy. (Most psychologists have no training in the practice of medicine and they cannot prescribe medications or order laboratory tests.) Doctoral-level psychologists must go on to complete a year of postgraduate training (called an *internship* or sometimes a *residency*) in which they gain practical experience in assessing patients and doing therapy in order to be able to treat patients. There is no national accrediting body for psychologists, but most states require psychologists to be licensed in order to see patients. Typical licensure requirements include passing a written and sometimes an oral examination and having completed a degree and an internship in a program approved by the American Psychological Association.

Many, perhaps even most, psychotherapists have a degree in social work, a field that emphasizes the interactions of individuals with their various social groups: their family, community, and culture. A *clinical social worker* specializes in helping individuals, couples, or families with emotional or relationship problems by means of counseling and psychotherapy. Most clinical social workers have a master of social work degree (M.S.W.), though some have a doctoral-level degree (D.S.W. or Ph.D.). Like psychologists, social workers must be licensed in the state where they practice, and licensure typically requires an approved degree, professional references, and, often, passing an examination. Social workers may apply for membership in the Academy of Certified Social Workers of the National Association of Social Workers, if they have a master's degree in social work from an approved program, have completed two years of social work experience that has been supervised, have submitted professional references, and have completed a written examination. The letters A.C.S.W. in a social worker's title indicate this membership. A more advanced certification is the Diplomate in Clinical Social Work, requiring more years of experience and a more advanced examination. These social workers use the designation D.C.S.W. to indicate this certification. The American Board of Examiners in Clinical Social Work is another organization that issues a certification in advanced practice to social workers who have a master's degree in clinical social work from an approved college or university program, have practiced in the field for five years and seen clients under supervision for a certain number of hours, and have had colleagues and supervisors attest to their competency. Clinical social workers with this certification add the designation B.C.D. after their name.

Some psychiatrists decide to limit their practice to psychotherapy and become primarily psychotherapists, though this is becoming increasingly rare. Individuals with degrees in nursing may work as psychotherapists. Often they have taken advanced training in therapy to do so.

Some psychotherapists have a degree in counseling and have trained specifically in this field. *Counseling* differs from psychotherapy in its emphasis on giving advice and guidance rather that treating disorders. School counselors often have this kind of training background. Though there is certainly a lot of overlap, counseling can be thought of as helping psychologically healthy individuals to improve and enhance their functioning and coping skills, and psychotherapy as treating individuals with psychological problems and returning them to normal functioning. Clergy may get training in pastoral counseling and even advanced training in psychotherapy. Pastoral counselors, of course, usually emphasize spiritual growth, and the religious and ethical principles of their religious background will guide their work with clients. The National Board of Certified Counselors offers a variety of certifications in counseling to individuals with a variety of educational backgrounds.

There are several medical professionals who are trained to work in conjunction with and under the direct supervision of physicians. The *physician's assistants* (P.A.) and *nurse practitioner* are "physician extenders" who see patients and are permitted in some states to prescribe medications. These professionals are most frequently encountered in primary care settings: family practice, obstetrics and gynecology, and some surgical practices, where they can perform more routine and uncomplicated aspects of care. They sometimes function in a similar capacity in busy mental health practices and clinics, where they may see patients for routine monitoring of established treatment plans. Depending on local regulations, physicians must sometimes be physically present in the same office suite and review and sign off on the work of these professionals within twenty-four hours.

Of all these professionals, the one with the most training and experience in the treatment of persons with illnesses is the psychiatrist. I'm hard pressed to think of a reason why any parents who suspect serious depression in their child shouldn't *begin* the evaluation with a psychiatric consultation.

As with choosing any other physician, choosing a psychiatrist must usually start with a review of your medical insurance plan. Psychiatry is considered a specialty referral, and depending on your coverage, some phone calls and investigation will be necessary and will save a lot of headaches later. If your family is enrolled in a health maintenance organization (HMO), your child will only be able to see a psychiatrist approved by the plan and usually only with the referral of your primary care physician. If your family is covered by a preferred provider organization (PPO), the primary care referral may or may not be necessary and you may be able to go outside the organization's list of approved doctors for psychiatric care at a lower reimbursement rate (you will be required to pay for a higher percentage of the fee).

HMOs and PPOs frequently "outsource" their mental health services. This usually involves contracting with a particular mental health practice or other provider group. Sometimes this group provides all the treatment services, sometimes it provides certain services and manages others, contacting other providers and approving treatment with them upon receipt of written treatment plans. (Chapter 17 goes into more detail on these insurance issues.)

More and more psychiatrists, especially child psychiatrists, are opting not to participate in insurance plans because of all the paperwork and other kinds of extra work involved in dealing with managed care organizations. These practitioners require their fees be paid in full at the time of each visit; patients must then submit receipts to their insurance plan and deal with the reimbursement issues themselves. Unfortunately for individuals needing care, oftentimes the best practitioners fall into this category, making for some difficult financial decisions.

Once you know what your options are from an insurance standpoint, you can narrow your decision-making. Pediatricians usually have a consultative relationship with a psychiatrist, or psychiatric practice, to whom they are confident referring their patients. This is perhaps the best referral source. If you live in a community where there is a university with a medical school, the medical school will have a department of psychiatry and usually a practice affiliated with the faculty.

Many psychiatrists who are competent in caring for adolescents with mood disorders are not child psychiatrists, that is, they have not done a child psychiatry fellowship in addition to their general psychiatric training. As I've noted previously, caring for an adolescent with a mood disorder is in many cases more like treating an adult than treating a child. Psychiatrists who work well with adolescents often start out with a more general psychiatric practice in adult or child psychiatry, then gradually develop an adolescent practice because they enjoy working with patients in this age range and are good at treating adolescents. This is exactly the kind of psychiatrist you want for your child. Your pediatrician or family doctor, or perhaps a relative or friend who is a medical or mental health professional, or a member of the clergy may be helpful in your search.

Choosing a psychotherapist will involve much the same process. It may be easier, in fact, because psychiatrists almost invariably have working relationships with a number of psychotherapists to whom they refer their patients. Because the fees of nonphysicians are usually lower than psychiatrists' fees, paying "out-of-pocket" may be a bit more feasible. But remember that psychotherapy sessions are often weekly for many months, so the total outlay may be substantial. Given the devastating effects of untreated depression on the lives of adolescents, this is clearly a good investment.

Another factor to keep in mind when going through this selection process is that the management of mood disorders is a long-term proposition. One of the most important requirements for successful treatment is a *long-term* relationship with the treatment professionals. I cannot emphasize this point strongly enough. One of your goals in selecting a professional is to find someone who will be providing care for *years* to come.

Do not be afraid to get a second opinion about treatment. When the patient doesn't seem to be benefiting from treatment, getting another clinician to take a fresh look at the diagnosis and treatment plan can be very helpful. The treating physician will not, or at least *should* not, object to a request for a second opinion. In fact, a physician often welcomes the opportunity to get some help and advice in managing a difficult case. Many university medical centers provide consultation services and often have mood disorder experts on the staff. The consultant will be able to help most if he or she can review as many treatment records as possible, so some advance work on your part in collecting records in preparation for a consultation is well worth the effort. The consultant's report usually has a "have you thought of . . . " tone and will often raise questions rather than answer them. But this is just what will be helpful for the clinician who already knows the patient well and will thus be able to incorporate new ideas into the treatment plan.

Beware, however, of the temptation to get too many opinions in a tough case. It is *not* useful to radically alter a treatment approach every month or

Figure 15-1 A sample treatment record. This sort of record is extremely helpful in recording medication response, especially when the mood disorder is difficult to treat and multiple medications have been tried. A more detailed form used by the Harvard Bipolar Group to chart treatment is available from www.manicdepressive.org/moodchart.html.

so based on yet another consultant's recommendation; a parade of experts can result in more confusion than clarity.

The treatment of mood disorders often must change and adjust to the clinical situation: medications are started and stopped, added and taken away; therapy may need to be more intense and frequent at times, and the patient may be able to take a "vacation" when things are going well. Especially for adolescents, who often have trouble expressing their feelings and who sometimes are just plain oppositional, having a psychiatrist and psychotherapist who know them well is a tremendous asset in their treatment.

Keep a treatment record for your child. This can be in chart form, as in figure 15-1, or simply a diary. Record what medications the adolescent has taken, including dates of starting and stopping, doses of medications, and blood levels (if they have been ordered). List any side effects or problems the youngster has had with the medications and also the treatment response. This sort of list is extremely useful in many different situations: if there is a change in doctors, if you request a second opinion, if treatment seems to have stalled for some reason and a detailed review of all treatments and responses to treatment is needed to see what hasn't yet been tried.

ELIMINATING PATHOLOGICAL INFLUENCES: MOOD HYGIENE

The word *pathological* is derived from the Greek word for "disease," and by *pathological influences* I mean factors in the patient's environment that make illness symptoms worse or more difficult to treat. Just as an adolescent with diabetes must make lifestyle changes (including dietary changes, such as what to eat and the timing of meals) as a part of controlling blood sugar, so an adolescent with a mood disorder must make lifestyle changes to have the best control of mood symptoms. Sometimes this means a minor adjustment, sometimes a major overhaul, but this is *not* an "optional" part of the recovery process.

What do I mean by *mood hygiene*? Simply put: practices and habits that promote good control of mood symptoms in persons with mood disorders. *Hygiene* is a word that we probably don't use as much as we should in medicine — and we certainly don't use it as much as we used to. Hygeia was the Greek goddess of health, the daughter (or in some versions of the story, the wife) of Aesculapius, the god of medicine.

Hygiene, or *hygienics*, is the science of *the establishment and mainte-*

Figure 15-2 Hygeia. *Source:* Courtesy of the National Library of Medicine

nance of health (as opposed to the treatment of disease) and concerns itself with conditions and practices that are conducive to health. The hygienic conditions and practices we think of today are usually related to cleanliness, but the word really has a much broader meaning. The Johns Hopkins University's School of Hygiene and Public Health (founded in 1916; now the Bloomberg School of Public Health), University of London's School of Hygiene and Tropical Diseases (1924), and other such institutions were founded to study methods for the *prevention* of disease and for promoting and improving the health of whole communities. Predating these was the Mental Hygiene Association, founded in 1909 by former asylum inmate Clifford Beers (who probably had bipolar disorder) and now called the Mental Health Association; its purpose is to promote emotional health and well-being and advocate for better and more available treatment for psychiatric illnesses.

Several areas of research on mood disorders, especially bipolar disorder, show just how important preventive measures can be for improving symptom control in these illnesses. Things like stress management and lifestyle regularity make a big difference.

One of the most astute students of the study of mood disorders, German psychiatrist Emil Kraepelin, noticed that early in the course of illness of his patients with mood disorders, their mood episodes often came on after a stressful event in their life. In his textbook of psychiatry, published early in the twentieth century, Kraepelin noted: "In especial, the attacks begin not infrequently after the illness or death of near relatives . . . Among other circumstances there are occasionally mentioned quarrels with neighbors or relatives, disputes with lovers . . . excitement about infidelity, financial difficulties . . . We must regard all alleged injuries as possible sparks for the discharge of individual attacks." Kraepelin was quick to point out that these events were triggers, not causes, and that "the real cause of the malady must be sought in permanent internal changes which . . . are innate." Kraepelin noticed, however, that later in the course of the illness, attacks occurred "wholly without external influences" and proposed that at this later stage "external influence[s] . . . must not be regarded as a necessary presupposition for the appearance of an attack."[1]

Research has shown that severe depressive episodes in many young persons are preceded by the death of someone close to them or by some other loss or difficulty. One study found a significant association between adolescent depression and repeated episodes of loss or significant separation during childhood. The most interesting finding of the study was the lack of an association between depression and only one episode of serious loss. *Multiple* events were necessary.[2] Studies on adults with bipolar disorder have shown that the initial and early mood disorder episodes are often related to psychological stresses, but that after several episodes, the illness can take on a life of its own and episodes are more likely to arise spontaneously.

These sorts of findings are quoted to support the idea of a *kindling* phenomenon in mood disorders: a match held to a pile of wood may start a small flame that quickly dies out; but if the process is repeated often enough, a fire is kindled and no more matches are needed. In a similar way, repeated episodes of psychological stresses, especially loss, set off a chain of events in vulnerable individuals (perhaps individuals who have inherited a genetic vulnerability to mood disorders) and an episode of depression results. An interesting parallel phenomenon is seen in animal experiments. An epileptic seizure can be triggered in an animal by applying a small electrical current to its brain. If this is repeated often enough, the animal will start having seizures even *without* the electrical stimulation: seizures have been *kindled*.

Another interesting parallel in animals can be demonstrated by repeatedly giving animals small doses of stimulants such as cocaine. Over time, animals become *more* rather than less sensitive to the stimulant, and repeatedly giving the same small dose causes *increasing* amounts of behavioral stimulation in the animal. A close examination of the brain cells of these animals, with and without the prolonged stimulant treatment, reveals that a certain gene that was not previously active has been turned on by the repeated stimulant exposure. This same gene can be made to turn on by stressing the animals (by depriving them of water, for example). This work with animals, showing that electrical and chemical stimulation as well as stress can bring about long-term changes in behavior (possibly through alterations in gene function), is thought by many experts to be highly relevant to the study of mood disorders.[3] The observation that anticonvulsant medications, which have "anti-kindling" effects, are highly effective in treating bipolar disorder is one piece of evidence cited in support of this line of thinking.

Several direct observations on patients indicate that kindling may occur in individuals with mood disorders. First, patients sometimes have more environmentally triggered mood episodes early in the course of their illness and more spontaneously occurring episodes later. Second, they sometimes have an acceleration in their illness as they age, with episodes occurring more and more frequently as time goes on. And third, mood episodes make patients more sensitive to stress and more likely to relapse than they might otherwise be. In a study of fifty-two adult patients with bipolar disorder followed up for two years, those who relapsed during the time of the study were much more likely to have experienced some stressful event. In this group of patients, those with a greater number of prior mood episodes were *more* sensitive to these stresses: they were more likely to relapse under stress and they relapsed more quickly.[4] The worsening of depressive illnesses as individuals age has been demonstrated in many studies.

Given the observations that (1) psychological stress can make a person with bipolar disorder more vulnerable to having a mood episode and (2) as the person has more and more episodes, the symptoms can be triggered by smaller and smaller amounts of stress and adversity, then (1) *preventing* relapses of depressive episodes is extremely important and (2) individuals with mood disorders need to work hard to minimize situations of emotional stress in their lives.

Preventing Relapse with Medication

After the development of antidepressant medications made the medical treatment of severe depression widely available in the 1960s, the question quickly arose of how long antidepressant medications should be prescribed. Although we do not have enough information yet to answer to this question definitively, the information we do have supports long-term treatment.

Studies in adults clearly indicate that an antidepressant medication that has been effective for an individual with a serious depression should be continued for at least twelve months. I tell patients and parents of patients that anyone who has had a serious depression that has responded to treatment with an antidepressant medication shouldn't even consider discontinuing the medication for at least a year. By that point, many individuals come to realize they had been more depressed and more severely depressed than they ever realized while they were in the grip of the illness. These are the individuals who had really never known what a normal mood was like before starting on medication. Not infrequently, these patients come to their appointment at the twelve-month point ready to plead with me to let them *continue* taking antidepressant medication. They never need to. I am only too happy to let individuals who have been helped by antidepressant medication take it for as long as they wish. I am convinced by my personal experience of treating many patients with mood disorders that every relapse of depression increases the chances of the illness becoming more difficult to treat. Research data clearly indicate that early-onset depression is a more severe illness. Some guidelines for the treatment of adults with depression recommend that individuals with the onset of severe depression before the age of 20 take medication indefinitely because of the higher probability of relapses.[5] Instead of asking "why should I continue taking antidepressant medication?" the question for individuals who have had a serious depression should probably be "why *shouldn't* I continue taking antidepressant medication?" Individuals who have a family history of either bipolar disorder or recurrent major depressive disorder are especially well advised to take this long view.

For individuals with bipolar disorder, the evidence for the necessity of long-term treatment with medication is much more compelling. Bipolar disorder, especially childhood- or adolescent-onset bipolar disorder, is clearly a relapsing illness that must be treated continuously and indefinitely to prevent the development of episodes.

Addressing Substance Abuse

The surest recipe for treatment failure in mood disorders is the continued use of intoxicating substances. There are many reasons why adolescents with mood disorders must not drink alcohol and must certainly not use marijuana or other drugs.

The first is that alcohol and many drugs have direct toxic effects on the brain. In the chapter on substance abuse, I mentioned that drugs such as ecstasy have been shown to kill neurons. We know that chronic alcoholics develop memory problems and the wide-ranging decline in all mental abilities that psychiatrists call dementia. These damaging effects are more significant in the developing brain (remember that neurons and their interconnections are still growing and developing in an adolescent's brain). Substance abuse in young people is thought to interfere with the brain's developmental process and may disrupt brain development in permanent ways that, currently, we can only guess at.

By altering the chemical functioning of the brain, substance abuse has effects on mood as well. Persons who abuse alcohol and individuals who are "crashing" from binges of cocaine or amphetamines can go through profound depressive episodes that seem to be directly related to the chemical effect of the intoxicating substances. It's thought that the "high" of getting intoxicated from alcohol or anything else results from a massive stimulation of the pleasure centers of the brain. These centers become exhausted and depleted of their chemical messengers because of this massive overstimulation, and this depletion is what is thought to result in the depressive crash and other mood changes that occur after intoxication.

Thus, for individuals undergoing treatment for mood disorders, getting intoxicated interferes with the therapeutic process to relieve depression or to stabilize mood. A simple way of thinking about this is that getting intoxicated depletes the chemicals that antidepressants are trying to boost. I tell patients that drinking or getting high when under treatment for depression is like punching holes in a bucket that you are trying to fill with water—continued substance abuse makes treatment for a mood disorder pretty pointless.

I truly believe that marijuana is the most harmful in this regard, because it is the most insidious. Because marijuana is slowly absorbed into the fat cells of the body and slowly released between episodes of "getting high," crashes into depression and obvious withdrawal symptoms are less apparent. It's as if the usual time line for these phenomena gets so stretched out as to become almost undetectable. I've seen many persons with depression in all age ranges who were convinced that marijuana had no effect on their mood and who refused to stop—and whose depressions never quite went into remission.

My biggest lesson in this regard was from a young adult who had severe depressions that only partially responded to aggressive treatment with medications. A combination of quite a few medications was the only approach that kept him out of the hospital, and he was nearly nonfunctional in his family life and was unable to work. Joe insisted that marijuana was the only thing that helped him feel better for a few hours, and he absolutely refused to give it up.

One day I stepped into the clinic's waiting area to ask Joe to come back to the interviewing room for his medication appointment, but I didn't see him among the patients waiting for their appointments. There was a young man with a neck brace who looked familiar, but I thought Joe must have stepped out to the rest room. I turned to the receptionist and asked if she knew where Joe had gone, and the young man with the neck brace stood up. It was Joe, looking so bright-eyed and energetic that I hadn't even recognized him. It turned out that Joe had been in a swimming accident that had injured him badly enough to put him in a rehabilitation hospital for nearly three months—long enough for the marijuana to get out of his system completely. His depression steadily improved over this period, and by the time he got out, most of his medications had been discontinued and he was taking only an antidepressant. We had both learned an important lesson about the connection between depression and substance abuse the hard way (though it was certainly a lot harder on Joe than on me).

Substance abuse is, in a way, a means of coping with adversity by retreating into getting high. As I said in chapter 11, substance abuse also has the effect of crowding out other activities like school and family life. Another activity it crowds out is emotional maturation. Learning how not to get caught takes the place of learning how to trust and be trusted. Learning how to find and secure a steady supply of alcohol or drugs takes the place of learning how to make and keep healthy relationships with peers. Planning for the next high takes the place of planning for the next five years. Every mental health professional who has worked with adolescents can tell you that adolescents who are substance abusers seem to stop maturing emotionally at the age they started using. A 19-year-old who is able to stop using alcohol or drugs may have the emotional development of a 13-year-old, if that's when he started using. Catching up from this "maturity deficit" can take several years and a lot of therapy.

The most difficult issue parents face in this regard is knowing how much intervention on behalf of a substance-abusing adolescent is helpful and how much is "enabling." The concept of *enabling* a substance abuser has developed out of the treatment literature on alcohol abuse and refers to helpful actions on the part of family members that turn out to sustain rather than help stop the substance abuse. The classic example is the wife of an alcoholic who calls her husband's boss to report that her husband is "sick" and won't be in to work, when he is actually hung-over from his latest alcoholic binge. Rather than helping her husband she is actually enabling him to escape the consequences of his alcoholism—consequences that could force him to face his problem and decide to get treatment. Parents must decide how much interceding on their child's behalf with school authorities, other family members, and even the police is helpful and how much is "enabling" their child to remain a substance abuser. Because adolescents have a difficult time appreciating the long-term consequences of their actions, this is an even tougher problem. At what point is "tough love" too tough? There are no easy answers. In his powerful account of his daughter's struggle with alcoholism, Senator George McGovern writes, "The trouble with waiting for people to 'hit bottom' is that they may do so only after they have destroyed their lives or the lives of others."[6] (More on this dilemma in the next chapter.)

Adopting a Lifestyle That Promotes Mental Health

Just as physical stress is to be avoided by persons with certain physical problems, psychological stresses need to be identified and addressed by individuals who suffer from mood disorders. Although most of us have very little control of when and how stress and conflict come into our lives, we sometimes do have *some* control, and we can learn how to better manage the stress and conflict we can't avoid—and here I will put in another plug for counseling and therapy. Serious, *vigorous* attention to whatever ongoing sources of serious stress there may be is very important in the management of mood disorders. It's no accident that family therapy is so often recommended as an adjunct treatment in adolescent mood disorders. Numerous clinical studies show that ongoing family conflict is a major risk factor for relapse of depressive disorders in adolescents.[7] Relationship difficulties, too much advanced course work at school, an overly ambitious schedule of extracurricular activities—all these things can make for too many demands, too much stress, and can be risk factors for relapse of the mood disorder.

Adolescence is a time of developing lifestyle habits that will last a lifetime. Putting things off until the last moment invariably raises stress levels. Eliminating procrastination as a way of dealing with things goes a long way towards eliminating a lot of stresses. A growing body of research supports the notion that external regulators like regular sleep and activity schedules help with mood stability. *Establishing and sticking to a personal schedule* is very important. Establishing regular times for going to bed and getting up in the morning—seven days a week if possible—is highly recommended. Research on sleep shows that many other lifestyle factors contribute to or detract from good sleep. Consider cutting caffeinated beverages out of the diet completely, or at least make a habit of not drinking caffeine-containing soft drinks or coffee or tea after noon. Heavy meals late in the day should be avoided. Regular exercise has been shown to benefit sleep and has many other benefits besides, on blood pressure, for example. These factors are even more important for adolescents with mood disorders because of possible medication side effects on appetite and energy level. Several medications increase appetite and can be mildly sedating at first. Attention paid to healthy diet and exercise habits will go a long way towards improving energy level and avoiding unwanted weight gain. Consultation with a nutritionist can be very helpful, and developing an exercise program through the physical education department at school is often an option.

Many colleges and universities have added fitness centers to their athletic program's usual focus on team athletics.

It is impossible in these few paragraphs to distill this process of taking stock of personal conflicts and stresses and to detail the kind of individual attention it takes to deal with them. There's no list of helpful hints or dos and don'ts that I can give you here. Rather, I am recommending *serious examination and fundamental change*. This may involve something as minor as cutting back on participation on a team or as major as changing schools. Adolescents face many important decisions: decisions about selecting a high school and a college, after-school jobs and career paths, and for older adolescents, moving away from home and sometimes even getting married. These decisions need to be considered even more thoughtfully and carefully for those with a mood disorder. Counseling and psychotherapy are an invaluable help in sorting through options and making these decisions.

CHAPTER 16

The Role of the Family

When a child is miserable, parents want to make things better. Small children aren't very hard to cheer up. They will delight in a little toy surprise, a trip to a fast-food restaurant, helping mom or dad in the kitchen or with washing the car. But when an adolescent is seriously depressed, no amount of cheering up can help. Worse, when the symptoms of depression take the form of oppositional behavior and irritability, parents may discover that their child has become a hostile stranger who seems intent on tearing the family apart. Parents may be frightened and angered to discover that their son or daughter is drinking, using drugs, or engaging in other dangerous behavior. It's easy to be so paralyzed by fear and anger that ordinary decisions become overwhelming.

As in any illness, the role of the family includes support, understanding, and encouragement of the person who is ill, and the role of the parent includes nurturing, protecting, and supervising. The first step in being able to provide this kind of support is understanding some very important facts about the illness. It's also important to get the help and support *you* need to be there and be strong for your child.

RECOGNIZING SYMPTOMS

Never forget that someone with a mood disorder does not have control of his mood state. People who do not suffer from a mood disorder sometimes expect the person who does to be able to exert the same control over his emotions and behavior that they themselves are capable of. When we sense that we are letting our emotions get the better of us and we want to exert some control over them, we tell ourselves things like "snap out of it," "get a hold of yourself," or "pull yourself together." We are taught that self-control is a sign of maturity and self-discipline. We are indoctrinated to think of people who don't control their emotions very well as being immature, lazy, self-indulgent, or foolish. But you can only exert self-control if the control mechanisms are working properly, and in someone with a mood disorder, they are not.

People with mood disorders cannot "snap out of it," as much as they would like to (and it's important to remember that they want *desperately* to do so). Telling a depressed adolescent something like "pull yourself together" is simply cruel; in fact, it may reinforce the feelings of worthlessness and guilt and failure already present as symptoms of the illness.

The first challenge facing family members is to change the way they look at behaviors that might be symptoms of the illness—behaviors like not wanting to get out of bed, being irritable and short-tempered, or being "hyper" and reckless or overly critical and pessimistic. Our first reaction to these sorts of behaviors and attitudes is to see them as laziness or meanness or immaturity and to be critical of them. In a person with a mood disorder, this almost always makes things worse: criticism reinforces the depressed adolescent's feelings of worthlessness and failure, and it alienates and angers the hypomanic or manic individual.

This is a hard lesson to learn: don't always take behaviors and statements at face value. Learn to ask yourself, before you react, "Could this be a symptom?" Little children frequently say "I hate you" when they are angry at their parents, but parents know that this is just the anger of the moment talking and that these are not their child's true feelings. Irritable, depressed adolescents will say "I hate you" too, but this is the illness talking, an illness that has hijacked their emotions. The depressed adolescent might also say, "It's hopeless, I don't want your help." Again, this is the *illness* and not your child rejecting your concern.

GETTING INVOLVED IN TREATMENT

Because adolescence is, by definition, a time of transitioning from childhood to adulthood, it's sometimes difficult for parents to know how much involvement in their child's treatment is appropriate. Legally, parents must usually give consent for the treatment of a child under 18, though some states allow younger adolescents to legally consent to mental health and substance-abuse treatment. Parents have a right to ask questions and get answers about their child's treatment, but psychological treatment is always predicated on the assumption that the patient's sessions with the therapist are private. Most clinicians lay out ground rules about these privacy issues at the beginning of treatment.

Therapists will always break confidentiality if dangerous behavior is at issue and in some other compelling situations where the patient's best interest is served by doing so, but parents must be able to trust that a certain amount of confidentiality is appropriate and helpful in the adolescent's treatment. Having a "right" to information doesn't mean it's always right to ask for it. Insisting on hearing the details of therapy sessions from the therapist (or the child) is counterproductive.

Don't ask the therapist or psychiatrist to confront your adolescent about behaviors you've observed if you can't be there to back up your observations. I find that separate conversations with the patient and the parents about these sorts of issues often become "yes, he did—no, I didn't" sessions that are simply not helpful for anyone. Going along with your child to doctor's appointments and sharing your observations and concerns during the visit *in the child's presence* eliminates miscommunication and ensures that everyone—therapist, parents, and patient—is operating with the same set of information.

Above all, do not call the therapist or psychiatrist and say, "I don't want my child to know that I called you, but I think it's important to tell you that . . ." There's nothing more infuriating or demeaning than to have someone sneaking around reporting on you behind your back. Adolescents are exquisitely sensitive to issues of trust and will not benefit from treatment with someone they believe is allied with their parents and "against" them. Don't ask the psychiatrist or therapist to keep secrets.

Parents can also, however, err on the side of not being involved enough in their child's treatment, for fear of being a "tattle-tale"; they assume the clinician will notice the same things they've noticed about changes in moods or behaviors. One of the most valuable ways a family member can help in treatment is to provide a clear, undistorted view of the situation to the clinical team treating the adolescent. In my experience, family members are frequently the first to pick up on subtle changes in behaviors and attitudes that signal the beginnings of a relapse. I don't know how many times I have seen a patient in the clinic or even in the emergency room who has reassured me that she is feeling fine, whose behavior and mood seem normal, whom I send on her way, making a note in the chart that she is doing well, only to receive a panicked phone call from a parent or other relative a few hours later. "Didn't she tell you that she's lost ten pounds?" ". . . hasn't slept in three nights?" ". . . got suspended from school?" Contrary to popular belief, psychiatrists cannot read minds! Communicate your concerns openly and sincerely and supportively—almost anything that might otherwise seem intrusive can be forgiven.

Don't ask the psychiatrist or therapist to make parental decisions, and don't abdicate parental authority to the treatment team. The professionals are there to make recommendations and suggestions but not to make family decisions. Saying something like "you can't go to Tampa on spring break because the doctor said you can't" gives the adolescent the message that the parent has ceded authority to the professionals or, even worse, is incompetent to make decisions. It may cut off debate and argument in the short run but will inevitably backfire, actually encouraging defiant behavior. Remember that one of the goals of family therapy is to clarify roles and *your* parental authority. Adolescents need to know and to feel that their parents are in charge in the home.

Your goal is to have your child trust you when she feels most vulnerable and fragile. She is already dealing with feelings of deep shame, failure, and loss of control related to having a psychiatric illness. Be supportive, and yes, be constructively critical when criticism is warranted; but above all, be open and honest and sincere.

SAFETY ISSUES

Never forget that mood disorders can occasionally precipitate truly dangerous behavior. The dark specter of suicidal violence haunts those with serious depression, and the rageful irritability of mania can lead to frightening assaultive behavior. Violence is often a difficult subject to deal with, because the idea is deeply embedded in us from an early age that violence is primitive and uncivilized, a kind of failure or breakdown in character. Of course we recognize that the person in the grip of psychiatric illness is not violent because of some personal failing, and perhaps because of this, people sometimes hesitate to admit the need for a proper response to a situation that is getting out of control: when there is some threat of violence from the adolescent, towards himself or others.

Although family members cannot and should not be expected to take the place of psychiatric professionals in evaluating suicide risk, it is important to have some familiarity with the issue. As I've already mentioned, youngsters who are starting to have suicidal thoughts are often intensely ashamed of them. They often hint about "feeling desperate," about not being able to "go on," but may not verbalize actual self-destructive thoughts. It's important not to ignore these statements but rather to clarify them. Don't be afraid to ask, "Are you having thoughts of hurting yourself?" People are usually relieved to be able to talk about these feelings and get them out in the open where they can be dealt with. But they may need permission and support in order to do so.

Remember that the period of recovery from a depressive episode can be a time of especially high risk for suicidal behavior. People who have been immobilized by depression sometimes develop a higher risk for hurting themselves as they begin to get better and their energy level and ability to act improve. Also, patients having mixed symptoms—depressed mood and agitated, restless, hyperactive behavior—may be at higher risk of self-harm. In fact, there is some evidence that mixed, or dysphoric, mania is the most dangerous mood state in this regard.[1]

Another factor that increases the risk of suicide is substance abuse, especially alcohol abuse. Alcohol not only worsens mood, it lowers inhibitions. People do things when drunk that they wouldn't do otherwise. Increased use of alcohol increases the risk of suicidal behaviors and is definitely a very worrisome development that needs to be confronted and dealt with.

The development of serious suicidal risk calls for action. Have an emergency plan and be prepared to use it. Don't hesitate to invoke involuntary commitment procedures if you are really worried and your child is not cooperating with the need for evaluation.

A less frequent but nevertheless very real risk of violence is the violence towards others that can occur in mood disorders. Friends and family members should not hesitate to call for police help if they feel threatened. "What will the neighbors think?" should not be a concern where safety issues are concerned. If the situation is becoming dangerous, don't call the psychiatrist's office or the local emergency room—dial 911. Police officers are accustomed to dealing with psychiatrically ill individuals. They know safe physical restraint techniques, and they will be familiar with psychiatric emergency services in the community. In my experience, police officers will have the same goals you do in the situation: transporting the individual quickly and safely to the appropriate health care facility so that he can receive proper treatment.

ARRANGING HOSPITALIZATION AND INVOLUNTARY TREATMENT

Every community has laws and procedures to safeguard individuals who are unable to care for themselves. Laws allowing the removal of children from the care of parents who are abusing them are the most obvious example. Another set of laws allows the treatment of individuals for psychiatric illnesses against their will in certain circumstances. One of the most difficult things parents might be called on to do for their child with a mood disorder is to sign for hospitalization over the child's protest or to initiate involuntary treatment or commitment.

The laws governing the admission of minors to psychiatric facilities and the involuntary commitment laws for adults are usually state laws and so vary from one state to another; in addition to these state-by-state variations, local procedures can vary from community to community. This means that I can't provide a step-by-step procedure here, only general principles—but in my experience, it's not the procedures that confuse people but the general principles, so I think a brief discussion of this matter is worthwhile.

Parents can consent to psychiatric hospitalization for their minor child in many jurisdictions, but there is often a judicial review of some kind to protect the rights of the minor. This process is to prevent a parent from dealing with a troublesome child by simply signing him or her into a psychiatric hospital. Thus, the admission of a minor to a psychiatric hospital, though sometimes technically a "voluntary" procedure, might involve a judicial hearing similar to those held in the case of involuntary commitments (sometimes this is true even if the adolescent is willing to be in the hospital).

Law and legal procedures governing the provision of psychiatric treatment (or any kind of medical treatment for that matter) against a person's stated wishes are based on the knowledge that, first, an individual whose judgment is immature and unformed cannot make sound decisions about medical treatment and, second, an adult whose judgment is clouded by the symptoms of an illness often does not make the same decisions about treatment that he would make if his judgment were not impaired. The delirious motor vehicle accident victim who has suffered massive blood loss may moan "I want to go home" as he loses consciousness on the stretcher, but the ER team will ignore such a statement and proceed to do what they have to do to save the person's life. It is presumed that if the person were alert and thinking clearly and understood the implications of "going home," he would not make such a request. No one would ask a screaming toddler for written permission for a needed blood test. Similar principles underlie psychiatric commitment law: treatment is given to persons against their will if immature or clouded judgment prevents them from making good decisions about their treatment. Minors fall into this category. Depressed older adolescents may feel so hopeless that they think treatment has no chance of helping. Thinking processes in mania can be so disorganized and scattered that seeking out and cooperating with treatment is not possible. In either case, there are mechanisms to get needed treatment for persons whose immaturity or psychiatric symptoms blind them to the need for it.

Fortunately, these laws also have safeguards built in to prevent confinement in a psychiatric hospital for the wrong reasons. Decades ago, it was very easy to invoke commitment law and often required only the signature of a relative or family physician to hospitalize a person for weeks or months, even years. People were hospitalized for all kinds of bogus reasons, and serious abuses of individual rights occurred. Laws became much stricter in the 1960s and 1970s to prevent these abuses. The main change was the addition of *dangerousness* as a commitment criterion. Unless an individual's behavior is truly dangerous to self (usually meaning suicidal behavior) or others, he or she cannot be committed for involuntary psychiatric treatment. In the case of minors, the need for and appropriateness of the level of treatment are the sorts of criteria used.

Requests or petitions for psychiatric hospitalization do not necessarily mean that the person who is alleged to be psychiatrically ill will be hospitalized. Parents cannot simply sign a child into a facility; only a doctor can admit someone to a hospital. A parent's request for admission or involuntary commitment usually allows the youngster to be transported to an emergency room, where a physician will make a decision about hospitalization. The child may be released if she does not meet legal criteria for admission or commitment.

Involuntary commitment is a very serious legal procedure in which an individual is confined against his or her will and temporarily loses some rights of self-determination. For this reason, the law and the courts take involuntary psychiatric treatment very seriously, and many safeguards against abuses are built into the procedures. The person requesting an involuntary commitment must usually appear at the local courthouse or police station to give information and, in some jurisdictions, must make a sworn statement before a judge or magistrate. Parents will be asked for specific and detailed information about their child's behaviors. This is often frustrating for those trying to get help for their loved one. They may feel that being asked a lot of questions is uncaring or that someone is questioning their judgment or their motives. It's important to remember that in the days when individuals could be confined to psychiatric hospitals simply because a relative or doctor "thought it was best" for them, significant abuses of civil rights resulted. With serious attention on the part of the issuing magistrate or judge to documenting the facts and a close questioning of the need for psychiatric admission for minors and involuntary treatment of adults, we know the system is working.

Some form of judicial review (a "commitment hearing") occurs at some point in the process (usually a few days after hospitalization), at which a judge or hearing officer determines that the admission procedure was done properly and legally. Although this is a legal proceeding, it is not a big courtroom scene. Usually a conference room in the hospital is used, only a few people are present, and the proceedings are kept confidential (not a matter of public record). The patient is allowed legal representation—in fact, an attorney will be appointed if the patient does not have one. As noted above, in some jurisdictions, even when both parents and child agree to hospitalization, a similar hearing occurs to safeguard the rights of the minor.

Involuntary commitment for psychiatric treatment does not usually affect people's other legal rights. Wills or other legal instruments they have executed are not invalidated, and patients do not become legally "incompetent" in other areas. Hospitalization and treatment are the only issues that are addressed in commitment hearings.

I am aware that the topic I'm discussing here is very frightening. It might seem that a person's liberty and the right of self-determination can be taken away all too easily. At the risk of sounding glib, however, I want to reassure readers that involuntary commitment of an individual is *not* a quick and easy procedure. On the contrary, in my experience, most people are surprised at how difficult it is to invoke these laws, how many safeguards are built into the procedures, and how seriously the strict interpretation of the laws is taken by everyone involved. These laws have been carefully written in the interest of helping, not simply confining, people with severe psychiatric illnesses. In my experience, they are effective at doing just that.

GETTING THE SUPPORT *YOU* NEED

It is important that family members recognize their own need for support, encouragement, and understanding in dealing with adolescent mood disorders. Mental health professionals go home every day and leave behind their work of dealing with psychiatric illnesses, an option that most parents and other family members do not have. Dealing with a seriously depressed adolescent day after day and living with a frequently irritable, cranky teenager can be frustrating and exhausting. The changes and unpredictability of the moods of someone with a mood disorder intrude into home life and can be the source of severe stress in family relationships, straining them to the breaking point.

Perhaps the most difficult challenge is that posed by an adolescent with a mood disorder who is consistently resistant to getting treatment. The most astonishing learning experience for medical students and interns is encountering their first patient who repeatedly refuses to continue with a treatment that will keep him well and is, often, the only way to avoid hospitalization. I remember as a resident reading the chart of an adult patient with bipolar disorder who had been admitted to the hospital dozens of times after stopping lithium, and wondering what on earth would make a person make such a foolish decision again and again. I remember thinking that taking three capsules of lithium a day seemed a very small inconvenience compared with spending what added up to several years of this patient's life in a psychiatric hospital. I've since learned that making peace with having this illness and staying in treatment is much more difficult than healthy people realize. And it is even more difficult for individuals who must start taking medications at an age when none of their peers have to bother with such things—when the only people they know who take medication are "old people" and "sick people." It's very difficult for a young, physically healthy person who's feeling well to take medication every day. The idea of taking medication to control one's moods and mental processes is also daunting.

But the harder lesson for parents is learning that there is no way that anyone can *force* an individual, even one's own child, to take responsibility for treatment. Unless the individual makes the commitment to do so, no amount of love and support, sympathy and understanding, cajoling or even threatening can make someone take this step. Even parents who understand this at some level may feel guilty, inadequate, and angry at times, dealing with this situation. These are very normal feelings. Parents should not be ashamed of these feelings of frustration and anger but rather get help with them.

But even when the adolescent does take responsibility and is trying to stay well, relapses can occur. Family members might wonder what *they* did wrong. Did I put too much pressure on her? Could I have been more supportive? Should I have been tougher and set firmer limits? Why didn't I notice the symptoms coming on sooner and get her to the doctor? A hundred questions, a thousand "if only's." Another round of guilt, frustration, and anger.

On the other side of this issue is another question: how much understanding and support for the adolescent with a mood disorder might be *too* much? What is protective and what is overprotective? Should you call your child's coach with excuses as to why she isn't at practice? Should you pay off credit card debts from hypomanic spending sprees caused by dropping out of treatment? When an irritable outburst ruins a family occasion, should the teenager be grounded for her behavior? I've already discussed the concept of "enabling" a substance abuser to continue abusing by shielding him from the consequences of his problem. The same dynamic can operate even when substance abuse is not at issue. What actions constitute helping a sick person, and what actions are helping a person to be sick? These are thorny questions and complex issues. To say that they have no easy answers sounds pat and rather feeble, but it is frustratingly true. Punishing the teen for symptoms like irritability and low energy and motivation isn't fair, but not holding the teenager accountable for *any* of her actions isn't helping her either. Clearly, putting the adolescent too much in charge of her treatment is not right, but letting her have no say in treatment decisions isn't right either. Parents need a forum to process their decisions and strategies; by walking through their successes and failures with experienced peers or a professional, they can learn from them. You will need and deserve a lot of support and encouragement for the tough work of helping with these illnesses—just for hanging in there, every day, day after day.

For all these reasons, it's vital that family members seek out support groups and organizations and consider getting counseling or therapy for themselves to deal with the stresses caused by these illnesses. Like many chronic illnesses, mood disorders afflict one but affect many in the family. It's important that *all* those affected get the help, support, and encouragement they need.

CHAPTER 17

Planning for Emergencies

T he decisions we are forced to make in a crisis situation are frequently
not the decisions we would make under other, calmer circumstances. When an emergency arises for which we are unprepared,
we are usually forced to make up our response as we go along. One of the
best ways to prepare for an emergency is to have a crisis plan ready to go.

Because so many highly effective treatments are available for a mood
disorder, we sometimes forget that this is a potentially fatal illness. And in
dealing with a disease that has the potential to become life-threatening, the
last thing you want is an improvised response to an emergency situation.

The frustration in the nurse's voice was apparent as she spoke into the emergency room phone.

"I hear you, Mrs. Winters, but the magistrate won't approve a petition for
involuntary treatment because you think she needs treatment. I need more information before we can—"

Suddenly, she put down the phone. "I can't believe it, she hung up on me!"
Susan looked down at her note pad and then turned to me. "Does the name
Anne Winters mean anything to you? That was her mom. She wanted someone to come out to their house and bring Anne into the emergency room. She
said the girl might be suicidal."

"The name doesn't ring any bells with me," I replied. "Let's try the computer
to see if she's ever had any treatment here before; maybe we've got some

records. Then we can try calling Mrs. Winters back." As Susan stepped over to the emergency room's computer terminal, I glanced at my watch. It was almost noon and I had a lunchtime lecture to give. "Susan, I have to go and give my lecture to the medical students. If we have a chart on Anne, can you order it from medical records? I'll be back a little after one and we can see what we're dealing with and get back with Mrs. Winters."

It was just minutes past one when my beeper went off, with a message to call the emergency room.

"Frank, this is Susan. Mrs. Winters and her daughter are here in the ER. Well, that's not exactly true. Mrs. Winters is here, but Anne won't get out of the car. Do you think you can come down?"

I hadn't done any parking-lot therapy for a while and, as I walked past the "Authorized Personnel Only Please" sign that marked the door to the emergency room, I wondered what I would find. Susan was waiting for me. "I went out and persuaded the girl to come in. They're in room five. Anne has secretly been making cuts on her wrist for several days, so I think she'll need to be admitted. I'll call the unit and see if we have any beds on the adolescent unit."

"How old is the girl? Has she been here before? Were you able to get some records?" I asked.

"She's sixteen and she was seen about two years ago in the emergency room. We should have the record soon, but the computer information shows that the discharge diagnosis from the ER was major depressive disorder."

"Well, that's some help. Let me go see them."

As soon as I opened the door to the interview room, I could see that (as usual) Susan had sized up the situation pretty accurately. Anne was a tall handsome girl dressed in baggy denim pants that looked to be at least four sizes too big, held up by bright yellow suspenders. She had a gray sweatshirt with sleeves so long that her hands were invisible. A few brownish smears on one of the sleeves must have been what clued Susan in to asking the girl about hurting herself. She was slumped in a chair in the corner of the room staring at the floor. Mrs. Winters was smartly dressed in a business suit, which made me think she had been at work before all this started. She didn't wait for me to ask a question to get started.

"The principal called me from school this morning and said Anne had told one of her friends she wanted to die. She's been staying with her father and me since spring break last week and is supposed to be going back to her mother and stepfather this evening. I could tell something was wrong with Anne, but her father's been gone on business for the past several days and I thought we'd talk to her together when he got back. This is a total shock to me. The school counselor suggested I call the doctor Anne was seeing, but when I did, I found out she's retired from practice. Then Anne tells me she hasn't taken her antidepressant for a month—I didn't even know she was on medication!"

Anne answered my questions with only angry glares, so I took Mrs. Winters to another office and let Susan try to sort out what had happened at school with the girl. It took a while to get Mrs. Winters calmed down, and even longer to get the whole story.

Anne's father had shared joint custody of the girl with his ex-wife since they had divorced about three years previously. He had married the present Mrs. Winters a year later. This Mrs. Winters knew nothing about Anne's mood disorder. She had gotten Anne to agree to come to the ER only by threatening to call the police, and she'd been worried the girl would jump out of the car the whole way downtown.

A phone call to Anne's father revealed that the girl had begun psychiatric treatment following the ER visit two years previously. She had started psychotherapy and some medication, and after a few months had recovered well from her symptoms. She was no longer in therapy but was supposed to be seeing the psychiatrist every month. I recognized the name of the psychiatrist as a colleague who had retired about three months earlier. I knew for a fact that she had sent letters announcing her retirement several months before she quit her practice group.

It turned out that when Anne ran out of medication, Mr. Winters had persuaded her pediatrician to continue it "until we can make other arrangements." That had been months ago, and Anne still didn't have a psychiatrist.

I heard a knock on the door. Susan peeked in. "Dr. Mondimore, can I see you for a moment?" "Excuse me," I said and stepped outside. Susan was holding the PPO and HMO list that was posted on the ER bulletin board. "Mr. Winters's medical insurance changed in April and the new plan doesn't pay here. If Anne needs to be admitted, she'll have to go to Harris Memorial."

As Susan filled in more details of Anne's history and suicidal thinking, it became clear that the girl would indeed need to be in the hospital. "Great," I grumbled. "Her step-mom had a terrible time getting her here. I don't think we should let Mrs. Winters transport the girl. Can you have the secretary call patient transportation and I'll call—" Susan's frown stopped me. "Our transportation won't take patients to a hospital outside our system. We'll need to call an ambulance."

"That will cost them several hundred dollars," I said. "We can't use our people for a three-mile ride?" Susan gave me her very best "I don't make the rules, I just follow them" look and said nothing. I took a deep breath and prepared to go in to tell the Winters that it would probably be several more hours before Anne could be admitted to a hospital.

People usually enjoy making plans—vacation plans, wedding plans, retirement plans. Planning for a psychiatric emergency is much less enjoyable, but, if you have a family member with a mood disorder, it is, unfortunately, much more important. Unlike with vacation plans, you won't be disappointed if you don't need to use these plans. But if you do need them, odds are you'll be very glad you made them.

It seems that Mr. Winters was operating under the assumption that his daughter's mood disorder was an easily treated problem that didn't require a specialist. As I've emphasized already, adolescent-onset mood disorders can be difficult to treat, and vigilance to signs of relapse is very important. Mr. Winters made a big mistake switching Anne's care to a busy pediatrician so soon after she had received her diagnosis and started treatment. Also, he and his new wife had obviously not had a discussion about Anne's mood disorder and what the step-mom should do if symptoms flared up. Mrs. Winters didn't know what to do or whom to call when Anne refused to come to the ER. Last but not least, the Winters were unfamiliar with their medical insurance plan requirements, so Anne wound up being taken to a hospital where their insurance would not approve hospitalization.

How long would it have taken to avoid all these mistakes? An hour or two? Maybe three? Obviously, this would have been time well spent.

KNOW WHOM TO CALL FOR HELP

Every person with a mood disorder should be under the care of a psychiatrist who is familiar with the patient's symptoms and course of illness. This means getting established with a new physician when your family moves to a new community or when any other event (such as the retirement of your psychiatrist) leaves your child "uncovered." Changes in insurance plans sometimes force a change in psychiatrist too. Don't put off making an appointment to get your child established as a patient in a new community or with a new practice. Because it can sometimes take months for records to be transferred from one office to another, ask for a copy of your child's records or a letter of introduction that you can take to the new doctor at the first appointment.

Also, be sure to inform your pediatrician or family doctor about your child's treatment for a mood disorder. The doctor should be told about the child's diagnosis and any medications the child is taking. If the child is taken to an emergency room or admitted to a hospital for *any* reason, be sure to have a list of medications he or she is taking available for the staff.

In choosing a new psychiatrist, don't hesitate to ask how the practice is covered after office hours. Also ask how easy it is to get a routine office appointment. Are appointment times set aside so that patients can get an appointment in a day or two for emergencies? Every psychiatrist or mental health clinic should have some means of seeing patients within twenty-four hours in cases of true emergency. Be sure you know how to contact the psychiatrist or the office at any time of the day or night and what arrangements are in place to handle emergencies. Does the psychiatrist see her own emergency patients, or does everyone in the practice rotate emergency "on-call" duty? The on-call system, though not ideal, is the standard in many communities, meaning your child may well see a doctor other than his regular one if there is an acute emergency. Are you prepared for such an arrangement, so that your child will be under the care of a psychiatrist who comes highly recommended?

Which hospital or hospitals does the psychiatrist or the practice have a relationship with? Is it the hospital you prefer? The hospital where your insurance covers inpatient psychiatric treatment? Some psychiatrists do not do inpatient work at all, that is, they do not secure admitting privileges to a hospital but refer patients who need hospitalization to colleagues who do. This is especially true of child psychiatrists. This means a loss of continuity of care and, sometimes, lost time while a new psychiatrist gets to know the patient. Ask about whether the psychiatrist cares for her patients in the hospital and, if not, to whom she refers her hospitalized patients.

If the answers to these questions are not satisfactory, consider your options. Ask your family doctor, family members, and friends for recommendations. Call the local chapter of the Mental Health Association, the National Depressive and Manic Depressive Association, or another advocacy group for a referral. (These groups are listed in Resources, following chapter 18.) Sometimes, your options are limited by medical insurance coverage—which brings us to another important aspect of being prepared.

INSURANCE ISSUES

Be familiar with the details of your medical insurance coverage of psychiatric illness. Unfortunately, most plans treat psychiatric illnesses differently from nonpsychiatric illnesses. For example, they frequently have different and stricter limits on hospitalization coverage, number of outpatient appointments they will pay for, and the percentage or amounts that patients must pay out-of-pocket for certain services ("copayments"). Some insurance plans exclude coverage for treatment of psychiatric illness altogether or provide psychiatric coverage for an additional charge.

Is there a lifetime "cap" on psychiatric services? This might be a limit on days of hospitalization or on number of outpatient appointments per year, or it might be a dollar-amount limit to coverage. Is your family limited to or covered at a lower rate at certain hospitals or practice groups? If your insurance company denies coverage for a hospitalization or for several days of hospitalization, what procedures must you follow to appeal the decision?

Hospital stays of all types are getting shorter, and psychiatric hospitalization is no exception. Hospitalization is reserved almost exclusively for life-threatening emergencies now, and patients are discharged as soon as possible. As a rule, patients are no longer hospitalized on a psychiatric unit or in a psychiatric hospital for weeks or months (an exception might be the inpatient treatment of a very malnourished patient with an eating disorder, and even these stays are becoming briefer). Does the psychiatrist have access to a *partial hospitalization* program? (Sometimes also referred to as a *day hospital*.) This alternative to traditional hospital treatment provides hospital-like monitoring and treatment during the day (or sometimes for only part of the day) but allows patients to return home in the evening and spend the night there. It is a very useful treatment option for mood disorders, because it offers a way to provide daily monitoring of mood symptoms and treatment response without the disruption to personal and family life that staying in a hospital causes. Some insurers cover a partial hospitalization (even insist on it), but others do not. Know where your insurance company and your psychiatrist stand on partial hospitalization.

Everyone these days seems to be talking about "managed care." If you are a member of an HMO, you are part of the managed care picture. (In a *health maintenance organization*, members pay a monthly fee to receive their medical care from the organization.) But even if you are not in an

HMO, aspects of managed care practice probably affect you in one way or another, no matter what kind of insurance you have.

Managed care means that the organization that is financially responsible for your child's medical care (your medical insurance company or HMO, for example) supervises or manages how much medical care he or she receives. This is accomplished in a variety of ways, some that may be visible to you, some not. The main purpose of this management is to minimize the use of more expensive types of medical care, usually meaning hospitalization and treatment by specialists. In an HMO, the patient may have to be referred by a primary physician to any specialists (including a psychiatrist) in order to be covered. Lab tests may be covered only if the primary physician approves of them (this can make getting the blood tests needed to monitor therapy with lithium and some other psychiatric drugs inconvenient).

Before a person can be admitted to a hospital, the physician often needs to get approval for hospitalization from the individual's insurance company, a process called *pre-admission review*. This consists of phoning an insurance company representative (usually a nurse or social worker) and giving the details of the clinical situation that justify a hospital stay. If this reviewer does not think a hospitalization is justified by the facts the physician relates, a doctor-to-doctor review is usually arranged. This pre-admission review can be a lengthy process and involve multiple phone calls to and from insurance company representatives and clinical staff. After the patient is admitted to a hospital, the treating doctor may be called every few days by someone from the HMO or from the insurance company asking why the patient still needs to be in the hospital, a function called *utilization review*. If this reviewer (usually a nurse) thinks your child should be discharged, she will tell your doctor (and you) that coverage will be denied after a certain date and that you will be financially responsible for any additional inpatient treatment. (A variety of appeals procedures usually kick in at this point if your doctor disagrees.) Once usually limited to inpatient treatment, managed care now monitors outpatient treatment as well, and psychiatrists are being asked to fill out forms specifying a treatment plan and requesting a certain number of office visits. All these hassles are the reasons why many psychiatrists who can afford to do so do not participate in managed care plans.

If the insurance plan includes coverage for pharmacy charges, you may not have a choice of brands of medication but will have to take whatever equivalent generic pharmaceutical the pharmacy stocks. Some HMOs have

Psychiatrist			
Name:	Business phone:	After-hours phone:	
Therapist			
Name:	Business phone:	After-hours phone:	
Pharmacy		Approved Hospital(s)	
Name:	Phone:	Name:	ER Phone:
Primary Care M.D.			
Name:	Business phone:	After-hours phone:	
Insurance Info.			
Policyholder:	Policy number:	Group number:	Pre-admission contact:

Figure 17-1 Medical information chart. Complete a chart or list with this information and keep it up to date.

expanded on this theme and limit coverage to certain medications belonging to a broadly defined class, not permitting their doctors even to prescribe others. (For a while, some insurers would not pay for SSRI antidepressants and would insist that tricyclic antidepressants be tried first.)

There was a time when medical treatment was controlled by doctors and patients. That time has passed. Managed care methods save millions upon millions of health care dollars. Some people argue that this means that more people have access to better medical care because the system is more efficient and effective. Others argue that *managed care* is an oxymoron. But whichever is the case, managed care methods are common in all types of insurance coverage now. Your type of medical insurance will almost certainly determine which hospital your child can be admitted to and may determine which doctor he or she can see. Your insurance company will probably supervise the length of any hospitalizations and control the number of office visits, and even which medications can be prescribed. All this means that you should closely scrutinize all aspects of insurance coverage for psychiatric illness—your existing policy and any new policies that you may have to choose from because of job changes. Don't put yourself in the position of getting an emergency room surprise.

Make a list of important phone numbers and other information. Some of the items you should include are shown in figure 17-1.

MORE ON SAFETY

The most dangerous emergency situation for adolescents with mood disorders, and one that frequently leads to hospitalization, is the development of suicidal thoughts and behaviors. As the parent of a depressed child, *never* lose sight of the fact that mood disorders are potentially fatal diseases.

No firearms should be kept in the home of an individual who has been seriously depressed. There are any number of scientific studies showing that having a firearm in a home increases the chances of a violent death occurring in that home, by either suicide or homicide.[1] For an illness whose symptoms can include suicidal depression and heightened irritability with loss of inhibitions, there is never, *ever* any justification whatsoever for having a gun of any type in the home.

The appearance of self-destructive thoughts and impulses is frightening both to the adolescent and to those around her. The tremendous stigma and disgrace that have been associated with suicide for centuries still make people reluctant to discuss these thoughts when they occur. These ideas, and notions like "only crazy people kill themselves," complicate what is really a much simpler clinical issue: suicidal thinking is a serious symptom of this illness; it must be evaluated quickly by a professional and must be managed swiftly and effectively. Individuals can be intensely ashamed of suicidal thoughts and feel that the development of self-destructive impulses is a kind of failure. It is not a failing in any way, of course, but a symptom of an illness. It is important to see the development of suicidal feelings in a depressed adolescent as a very dangerous symptom of serious illness, just like the onset of chest pains in someone with heart disease. When these symptoms occur, it's not time to wonder about what they mean, *it's time to call for help.* And just as with the development of chest pains in a heart patient, the development of suicidal feelings in a person with a mood disorder is often a reason for hospitalization.

Psychiatric hospitalization can be experienced as a terrible failure. Again, the clinical perspective tells us otherwise. Although we have gotten much, much better at treating mood disorders, our treatment methods are by no means perfect. Sometimes, despite everyone's very best efforts, relapses occur: the patient has serious symptoms such as suicidal feelings and requires hospitalization. When this happens, it's not time for self-blame or questions like "what did I do wrong?" Rather, it's time for healing.

One more reminder: serious depression can raise many issues of personal safety. These issues need to be anticipated, discussed, planned for, and promptly addressed if and when they occur.

CHAPTER 18

Looking Ahead

W e have made enormous progress in the last several decades in the field of psychiatry. The diagnosis of depression, bipolar disorder, and other psychiatric illnesses is much more accurate than it was even a decade ago, and the available treatments for these illnesses are far more effective than even a few years ago. But such advances have come about through trial and error, not because of a better scientific understanding of the causes of these diseases. We still do not understand what is "broken" in the nervous systems of individuals with psychiatric illness.

Thousands of scientists are now working on two great enterprises that will eventually lead to a fuller understanding of these illnesses and to new and more effective treatment approaches. The first of these is the field of neuroscience: the study of the biology and chemistry of the brain and nervous system. At the beginning of the twentieth century, physical and psychiatric examinations of patients with brain disorders followed by microscopic study of their brain tissue after death was the only available method to investigate diseases of the brain. Animal experiments conducted along similar lines complemented these studies, but this work resulted in only the vaguest outline of the organization of brain function. The locations of brain areas important for speech, movement, vision, and so forth, were discovered, but psychiatric illnesses remained so mysterious that ideas that had nothing to do with biology—theories such as psychoanalysis—were the only ones that seemed to offer any hope of understanding these problems.

Throughout the last century, however, breakthrough followed upon breakthrough, mostly in the field of the chemistry of brain functioning, as neurotransmitters were discovered, more powerful electron microscopes allowed the visualization of synapses and other cellular structures, and sophisticated chemical probes allowed scientists to work out the mechanisms by which neurons grow and communicate with each other. The discovery of G proteins inside the cells was another huge step forward, and new discoveries about the workings of the brain are being made every day.

Now, with new technologies for brain imaging such as PET scans (positron emission tomography) and SPECT (single photon emission computed tomography), scientists for the first time can see the brain at work in living persons. These imaging techniques can show changes in blood flow within the brain, locate areas that are hyperactive or abnormally low in activity, or detect abnormally high or abnormally low levels of brain chemicals such as serotonin and dopamine. This information is revealing the importance of the interplay of activity between different brain areas in the regulation of mood and is making it possible to identify the responsible circuitry. These techniques are allowing us to see how the brain of a person with a mood disorder functions differently from that of a person who does not have a mood disorder, and, perhaps even more interesting, what changes occur when a person receives treatment and is beginning to feel well again.

The second of these great scientific enterprises is the field of genetics. Here again, the development of new biochemical methods and molecular probes is what has made this research possible. The Human Genome Project and Celera Genomics recently announced that it had mapped almost all the genetic material in the human chromosomes. Although this is as yet a map with only a very few signposts and labels, discoveries of new genes are announced every day, and it is only a matter of time before the genetic mechanisms of mood disorders are unraveled. The identification of the genes that are associated with mood disorders is only one of the goals of work in this field. Just as important will be understanding the mechanisms by which genes turn on and off and other mechanisms that regulate the expression and work of the instructions encoded in the DNA molecule.

As the genetic basis of the mood disorders is discovered, we may find that our classification system for these disorders is all wrong and that we need a whole new diagnostic system for psychiatric illnesses that is based on which genes are involved in individual patients. Instead of *major depressive disorder* or *bipolar disorder II*, we may be diagnosing patients with something like *21q22 mood disorder*, a name derived from the location of a gene.

A new field within the larger one of genetics is that of *pharmacogenet-ics*. Rather than looking for genes that are associated with specific illnesses, this search is for genes that are associated with therapeutic response to par-ticular medications, an approach that promises to take the guesswork out of psychiatric therapeutics. A simple blood test may indicate which med-ication will work best for a particular patient, ending the lengthy and frus-trating trial-and-error approach we now must use in finding the right med-ication for an individual.

The two fields of neuroscience and psychiatric genetics are closing in on the causes and mechanisms of mood disorders from different directions. As these two enterprises advance, they will begin to inform each other— that is, advances in one field will lead to advances in the other. Discover-ing that a gene for a particular protein is associated with a particular mood disorder will tell neuroscientists that the protein is important in the regu-lation of mood. The discovery of some new enzyme in neurons that is im-portant in neuronal signaling will tell geneticists to focus on the gene for that enzyme in their linkage studies. Little by little, the whole picture will become clearer and clearer.

Advances in many seemingly unrelated fields hold promise for better un-derstanding of mood disorders, too: advances in computer technology, for example. Just as architects now use computers to visualize buildings before they are built, pharmacologists are using computers to visualize the three-dimensional structures of neurotransmitters, receptors, and pharmaceuti-cal agents to design new drugs. It is hoped that new pharmaceuticals that have a better "fit" with receptors or other targets will work faster, at lower doses, and with fewer side effects. Computers are also being used to model and study brain activity. Remember that the brain is much more than just a sophisticated computer: more like a network of millions and millions of individual computers. Advanced computers using *nonsequential neural ar-chitecture* to build *neural networks* (made up of many interconnected but independently computing units) show properties that would not be pre-dicted from known principles of computing. These properties are probably highly relevant to the study of human brain activity and psychiatric illness.

Our understanding of the biology of mood disorders is getting better all the time. With each advance we get closer to better diagnostic methods and safer and more effective treatments. The number of new medications con-tinues to grow, and many more new pharmaceuticals are "in the pipeline." With the more sophisticated use of nonpharmaceutical treatments such as transcranial magnetic stimulation, perhaps we'll be able to use lower doses of medications or help medications to work more quickly.

As we take the step from isolating genes to determining the function of those genes, we'll be able to design treatments more effectively and more rationally. This work also holds out the possibility of gene therapy: repairing the code in the DNA that causes mood disorders. The obstacles to be overcome before we can look for this type of cure can only be called daunting, even monumental. But scientists are closing in on these illnesses little by little, and with enough time and enough hard work, a cure might be possible.

As the mechanisms of illness development become known and the genetic vulnerabilities are identified, another exciting possibility emerges: prevention. Genetic data and a better understanding of what triggers the illness may allow the development of prevention programs aimed at averting illness development in individuals known to be at higher risk for a particular disorder.

People frequently ask me whether they or their child will have to take medication "for the rest of their life." I always tell them that no one knows the answer to this question because no one knows exactly what the treatment of mood disorders might be in the future. Physicians practicing in the 1930s probably could not have imagined that vaccines would one day almost eliminate diphtheria, polio, measles, and other childhood diseases, the common, often crippling, and sometimes fatal illnesses they saw so frequently in their patients but were so completely helpless to treat. The astonishing developments in neuroscience and genetics hold just this much promise for those afflicted with mood disorders. There is every reason to be hopeful that a time is not too far off when treatments for depression and other mood disorders will be more effective than *we* can now imagine.

Resources

SUGGESTED READING

Samuel H. Barondes, *Mood Genes: Hunting for the Origins of Mania and Depression* (New York: Oxford University Press, 1999).

> A clearly written and engrossing account of the tough science involved in the search for the genetic basis of mood disorders. An excellent introduction to the science of genetics.

Robert Hedaya, *The Antidepressant Survival Guide: The Clinically Proven Program to Enhance the Benefits and Beat the Side Effects of Your Medication* (New York: Three Rivers Press, 2001).

> An ambitious program for avoiding medication side effects that includes prescriptions for diet, exercise, and other lifestyle changes.

Kay Redfield Jamison, *An Unquiet Mind: A Memoir of Moods and Madness* (New York: Vintage Books, 1996).

> A powerful and moving narrative written with grace and wit by an international expert on bipolar disorder who suffers from it herself. A treasure of a book that contains some of the most engrossing and vivid descriptions of the experience of bipolar disorder ever written. A "must read" for anyone touched by bipolar disorder.

George McGovern, *Terry: My Daughter's Life-and-Death Struggle with Alcoholism* (New York: Villard Books, 1996).

> Senator McGovern's moving account of his daughter Terry's terrible and ultimately fatal addiction to alcohol cannot be too highly recommended for families dealing with an addicted relative. The senator vividly captures the dilemmas and struggles of a family trying to find the balance between helping their daughter without "enabling" her illness.

Francis Mark Mondimore, *Bipolar Disorder: A Guide for Patients and Families* (Baltimore: Johns Hopkins University Press, 1999).

> OK, so I'm a little biased about recommending this one, but I think it's a great resource for learning about bipolar disorder in all its variations. If you found the book you're holding in your hands helpful and want more information in the same style on bipolar disorder, this is your book!

Rolf Muuss, *Theories of Adolescence*, 6th ed. (New York: McGraw-Hill, 1996).

> This college textbook provides an excellent overview of adolescent psychology by means of well-written chapters on all the major psychological theories from G. Stanley Hall to Sigmund Freud to Erik Erikson and beyond.

William Styron, *Darkness Visible: A Memoir of Madness* (New York: Vintage Books, 1990).

> I recommend this book to medical students as one of the best accounts of the symptoms of depression available. A good book for family members to read to better understand the experience of serious depression.

SUPPORT AND ADVOCACY ORGANIZATIONS

All the following organizations provide information, educational resources, and often referrals to support groups and to clinicians in your community who are skilled in treating mood disorders. Get in touch with them all and become a member! In addition to the direct services they provide to consumers, these groups are active in combating the stigmatization of psychiatric illnesses, in advocating for better medical insurance coverage of psychiatric disorders, and in supporting research.

Depressive and Related Affective Disorders Association (DRADA)

> Meyer 3-181
> Johns Hopkins Hospital
> 600 North Wolfe Street
> Baltimore, MD 21287-7381
> 410-955-4647
> www.drada.org

National Alliance for the Mentally Ill (NAMI)

Colonial Place Three
2107 Wilson Blvd.
Suite 300
Arlington, VA 22201-3042
800-950-NAMI
www.nami.org

National Depressive and Manic-Depressive Association (NDMDA)

730 North Franklin Street
Suite 501
Chicago, IL 60610-7204
800-82-NDMDA
www.ndmda.org

National Foundation for Depressive Illness, Inc. (NAFDI)

P.O. Box 2257
New York, NY 10116
800-239-1265
www.depression.org

National Mental Health Association (NMHA)

1021 Prince Street
Alexandria, VA 22314-2971
800-969-NMHA
www.nmha.org

INTERNET RESOURCES

All the support and advocacy groups listed above have sites on the World Wide Web with links to many, many other useful resources. The astonishing range of resources on the Internet continues to grow, but remember that you'll also find inaccurate information, bias, and just plain nonsense on the Internet, and it's important to consider information sources very carefully. Here are a few more excellent resources.

American Academy of Child and Adolescent Psychiatry
www.aacap.org/

Information on child and adolescent psychiatry, including fact sheets for parents and caregivers.

Internet Mental Health
www.mentalhealth.com

> An excellent site, with information on many different disorders and their treatments, information on many psychiatric medications, and hundreds of reference articles from popular and professional publications.

Medscape
www.medscape.com

> This is primarily a news site for medical professionals, but it has a "patient information" section with many useful articles and links to other resources.

The Surgeon General of the United States
surgeongeneral.gov/

> Read the surgeon general's reports online, including comprehensive reports on child and adolescent mental health issues.

United States National Library of Medicine
www.nlm.nih.gov

> This site provides free access to Medline, the most comprehensive medical database in the world. You can access more than eight million references in thirty-eight hundred journals. An incredibly valuable resource.

WebMD Health
www.webmd.com

> A comprehensive and reliable source of health information. Thousands of pages on many different disorders, including depression, bipolar disorder, ADHD, eating disorders, and other illnesses. Includes an extensive on-line discussion group and regular "chats" on mental health issues.

Notes

PREFACE

1. D. Shaffer, P. Fisher, and M. Dulkin, "The Diagnostic Interview Schedule for Children Version 2.3: Description, Acceptability, Prevalence Rates and Performance in the MECA Study," *Journal of the American Academy of Child and Adolescent Psychiatry* 35, no. 11 (1996): 1427–39.

2. Peter Lewinsohn, Paul Rohde, John Seeley, Daniel Klein, and Ian Gotlib, "Natural Course of Adolescent Major Depressive Disorder in a Community Sample: Predictors of Recurrence in Young Adults," *American Journal of Psychiatry* 157, no. 10 (2000): 1584–91.

Chapter 1. DEPRESSION: SOME DEFINITIONS

1. William James, *The Varieties of Religious Experience* (New York: Penguin Books, 1982), 147.

2. William Styron, *Darkness Visible: A Memoir of Madness* (New York: Vintage Books, 1990), 58.

3. Johann Wolfgang von Goethe, *The Sorrows of Young Werther*, trans. Elizabeth Mayer and Louise Bogan (New York: Random House, 1971), 114.

4. Hugo Wolf quoted in Kay Redfield Jamison, *Touched with Fire: Manic-Depressive Illness and the Artistic Temperament* (New York: Free Press, 1993), 21.

5. Styron, *Darkness Visible*, 19.

Chapter 2. NORMAL ADOLESCENCE AND DEPRESSION IN ADOLESCENCE

1. N. Ryan, J. Puig-Antich, P. Ambrosini, H. Rabinovich, D. Robertson, B. Nelson, S. Iyengar, and J. Tomey, "The Clinical Picture of Major Depression in Children and Adolescents," *Archives of General Psychiatry* 44 (1987): 854–61.

2. Michael Rutter, *Changing Youth in a Changing Society: Patterns of Adolescent Development and Disorder* (Cambridge: Harvard University Press, 1980), 87.

3. Erik Erikson, *Childhood and Society*, 2d ed. (New York: Norton, 1963), 228.

4. Erik Erikson, *Identity, Youth, and Crisis* (New York: Norton, 1968), 131.

5. See James Marcia, "The Empirical Study of Ego Identity," in *Identity and Development: An Interdisciplinary Approach*, ed. Harke Bosma, Tobi Graafsma, and Harold Grotevant (Thousand Oaks, Calif.: Sage, 1994).

6. Rutter, *Changing Youth in a Changing Society*, 39.

7. Jerome D. Frank, *Persuasion and Healing: A Comparative Study of Psychotherapy*, rev. ed. (New York: Schocken Books, 1974), 316.

8. Ibid., 314.

9. Anna Freud quoted in Rolf E. Muuss, *Theories of Adolescence*, 6th ed. (New York: McGraw-Hill, 1996), 368.

10. Alfred Kinsey, Wardell Pomeroy, and Clyde Martin, *Sexual Behavior in the Human Male* (Philadelphia: W. B. Saunders, 1948), 639.

Chapter 3. THE MOOD DISORDERS OF ADOLESCENCE

1. P. Lewinsohn, H. Hops, R. Roberts, J. Seeley, and J. Andrews, "Adolescent Psychopathology I: Prevalence and Incidence of Depression and Other DSM-III-R Disorders in High School Students," *Journal of Abnormal Psychology* 102 (1993): 133–44.

2. Boris Birmaher, Neal Ryan, Douglas Williamson, David Brent, Joan Kaufman, Ronald Dahl, James Perel, and Beverly Nelson, "Childhood and Adolescent Depression: A Review of the Past 10 Years. Part I," *Journal of the American Academy of Child and Adolescent Psychiatry* 35, no. 11 (1996): 1427–39.

3. Douglas Williamson, Boris Birmaher, Barbara Anderson, Mayadah Al-Shabbout, and Ryan Neal, "Stressful Life Events in Depressed Adolescents: The Role of Dependant Events during the Depressive Episode," *Journal of the American Academy of Child and Adolescent Psychiatry* 34, no. 5 (1995): 591–98.

4. Ian M. Goodyer, "The Influence of Recent Life Events on the Onset and Outcome of Major Depression in Young People," in *Depressive Disorders in Children and Adolescents: Epidemiology, Risk Factors, and Treatment*, ed. Cecilia Ahmoi Essau and Franz Petermann (Northvale, N.J.: Jason Aronson, 1999), 241.

5. Birmaher et al., "Childhood and Adolescent Depression."

6. Ibid.

7. Elizabeth McCauley, Kathleen Myers, Jeffrey Mitchell, Rosemary Calderon, Kelly Schloredt, and Robert Treder, "Depression in Young People: Initial Presentation and Clinical Course," *Journal of the American Academy of Child and Adolescent Psychiatry* 32, no. 4 (1993): 714–22.

8. Birmaher et al., "Childhood and Adolescent Depression."

9. Maria Kovacs, Hagop Akiskal, Constantine Gatsonis, and Phoebe Parrone, "Childhood-Onset Dysthymic Disorder," *Archives of General Psychiatry* 51 (1994): 365–74.

10. Birmaher et al., "Childhood and Adolescent Depression."

11. Peter Lewinsohn, Daniel Klein, and John Seeley, "Bipolar Disorders in a Community of Older Adolescents: Prevalence, Phenomenology, Comorbidity and Course," *Journal of the American Academy of Child and Adolescent Psychiatry* 34, no. 4 (1995): 454–63.

12. William Coryell, Nancy Andreason, Jean Endicott, and Martin Keller, "The Significance of Past Mania or Hypomania in the Course and Outcome of Major Depression," *American Journal of Psychiatry* 144 (1987): 309–15.

13. G. Cassano, H. Akiskal, M. Savina, L. Musetti, and G. Perugi, "Proposed Subtypes of Bipolar II and Related Disorders: With Hypomanic Episodes (or Cyclothymia) and with Hyperthymic Temperament," *Journal of Affective Disorders* 26 (1992): 127–40.

14. See Sylvia Simpson, Susan Folstein, Deborah Meyers, Francis McMahon, Diane Brusco, and J. Raymond DePaulo, "Bipolar II: The Most Common Bipolar Phenotype?" *American Journal of Psychiatry* 150 (1993): 901–3.

15. Frederick K. Goodwin and Kay Redfield Jamison, *Manic-Depressive Illness* (New York: Oxford University Press, 1990), 69.

16. Hagop Akiskal, Jack Maser, Pamela Zeller, Jean Endicott, William Coryell, Martin Keller, Meredith Warshaw, Paula Clayton, and Frederick Goodwin, "Switching from 'Unipolar' to Bipolar II: An Eleven-Year Prospective Study of Clinical and Temperamental Predictors in 559 Patients," *Archives of General Psychiatry* 52 (1995): 114–23.

17. Lewinsohn et al., "Bipolar Disorders in a Community of Older Adolescents."

18. Hagop Akiskal, "The Prevalent Clinical Spectrum of Bipolar Disorders: Beyond DSM-IV," *Journal of Clinical Psychopharmacology* 16, suppl. (1996): 4S–14S.

19. Lewinsohn et al., "Bipolar Disorders in a Community of Older Adolescents."

20. Hagop Akiskal and Gopinath Mallya, "Criteria for 'Soft' Bipolar Spectrum: Treatment Implications," *Psychopharmacology Bulletin* 23, no. 1 (1987): 68–73.

21. Barbara Geller, Betsy Zimmerman, Marlene Williams, Kristine Bolhofner, and James Craney, "Bipolar Disorder at Prospective Follow-up of Adults Who Had Prepubertal Major Depressive Disorder," *American Journal of Psychiatry* 158 (2001): 125–27.

22. Barbara Geller, Kai Sun, Betsy Zimmerman, Joan Luby, Jeanne Frazier, and Marlene Williams, "Complex and Rapid-Cycling in Bipolar Children and Adolescents: A Preliminary Study," *Journal of Affective Disorders* 34 (1995): 259–68.

23. Rosalind Neuman, Barbara Geller, John Rice, and Richard Todd, "Increased Prevalence and Earlier Onset of Mood Disorders among Relatives of Prepubertal versus Adult Probands," *Journal of the American Academy of Child and Adolescent Psychiatry* 36, no. 4 (1997): 466–73.

24. American Academy of Child and Adolescent Psychiatry, "Practice Parameters for the Assessment and Treatment of Children and Adolescents with Bipolar Disorder," *Journal of the American Academy of Child and Adolescent Psychiatry* 36, no. 1 (1997): 138–57. Studies cited on page 140.

25. See Barbara Geller and Joan Luby, "Child and Adolescent Bipolar Disor-

der: Review of the Past 10 Years," *Journal of the American Academy of Child and Adolescent Psychiatry* 36, no. 9 (1997): 1168–76.

26. Geller et al., "Complex and Rapid-Cycling in Bipolar Children and Adolescents."

27. Emil Kraepelin, *Manic-Depressive Insanity and Paranoia*, trans. R. M. Barclay, ed. G. M. Robertson (Edinburgh: E. & S. Livingstone, 1921; reprinted New York: Arno Press, 1976), 1 (in reprint edition).

28. Joachim Puig-Antich, Joan Kaufman, Neal Ryan, Douglas Williamson, Ronald Dahl, Ellen Lukens, George Todak, Paul Ambrosini, Harris Rabinovich, and Beverly Nelson, "The Psychosocial Functioning and Family Environment of Depressed Adolescents," *Journal of the American Academy of Child and Adolescent Psychiatry* 32, no. 2 (1993): 244–53.

29. Paul Rohde, Peter Lewinsohn, and John Seeley, "Are Adolescents Changed by an Episode of Major Depression?" *Journal of the American Academy of Child and Adolescent Psychiatry* 33, no. 9 (1994): 1289–98.

30. Mark Sanford, Peter Szatmari, Miriam Spinner, Heather Munroe-Blum, Ellen Jamison, Christine Walsh, and Debbie Jones, "Predicting the One-Year Course of Adolescent Major Depression," *Journal of the American Academy of Child and Adolescent Psychiatry* 34, no. 12 (1995): 1618–28.

31. Maria Kovacs, Stana Paulaudkas, Constantine Gatsonis, and Cheryl Richards, "Depressive Disorders in Childhood III: A Longitudinal Study of Comorbidity and Risk for Conduct Disorders," *Journal of Affective Disorders* 15 (1988): 205–17.

32. Uma Rao, "Relationship between Depression and Substance Abuse Disorders in Adolescent Women during the Transition to Adulthood," *Journal of the American Academy of Child and Adolescent Psychiatry* 39, no. 2 (2000): 215–22.

33. Uma Rao, Neal Ryan, Boris Birmaher, Ronald Dahl, Douglas Williamson, Joan Kaufman, Radhika Rao, and Beverly Nelson, "Unipolar Depression in Adolescents: Clinical Outcome in Adulthood," *Journal of the American Academy of Child and Adolescent Psychiatry* 34, no. 5 (1995): 566–78.

Chapter 4. MOOD DISORDERS: A SUMMARY OF DIAGNOSTIC CATEGORIES IN THE DSM

1. American Psychiatric Association, *Diagnostic and Statistical Manual of Mental Disorders*, 4th ed. (Washington, D.C.: American Psychiatric Association, 1994), xvii. Note that epilepsy was considered to be a mental illness at the time.

2. Alfred Kinsey, Wardell Pomeroy, and Clyde Martin, *Sexual Behavior in the Human Male* (Philadelphia: W. B. Saunders, 1948), 639.

3. Douglas Williamson, Boris Birmaher, David Brent, Lisa Balach, Ronald Dahl, and Neal Ryan, "Atypical Symptoms of Depression in a Sample of Depressed Child and Adolescent Outpatients," *Journal of the American Academy of Child and Adolescent Psychiatry* 39, no. 10 (2000): 1253–99.

Chapter 5. MEDICATION ISSUES IN ADOLESCENCE

1. Nancy C. Andreason, *The Broken Brain: The Biological Revolution in Psychiatry* (New York: Harper and Row, 1985).

2. Roland Kuhn, "The Treatment of Depressive States with G 22355 (Imipramine Hydrochloride)," *American Journal of Psychiatry* 115 (1958): 459–64. This is an English translation of Kuhn's 1957 article.

Chapter 6. ANTIDEPRESSANT MEDICATIONS

1. Roland Kuhn, "The Treatment of Depressive States with G 22355 (Imipramine Hydrochloride)," *American Journal of Psychiatry* 115 (1958): 459–64.

2. C. K. Varley and J. McClellan, "Case Study: Two Additional Sudden Deaths with Tricyclic Antidepressants," *Journal of the American Academy of Child and Adolescent Psychiatry* 36, no. 3 (1997): 390–94.

3. J. Daly and T. Wilens, "The Use of Tricyclic Antidepressants in Children and Adolescents," *Pediatric Clinics of North America: Child and Adolescent Psychopharmacology* 45, no. 5 (1998): 1123–35.

4. Ibid.

5. C. K. Conners, "Methodology of Antidepressant Drug Trials for Treating Depression in Adolescents," *Journal of Child and Adolescent Psychopharmacology* 2 (1992): 11–22.

6. Rudolf Hoehn-Saric, John Lipsey, and Godfrey Pearlson, "A Fluoxetine-Induced Frontal Lobe Syndrome in an Obsessive-Compulsive Patient," *Journal of Clinical Psychiatry* 52 (1990): 343–45.

7. Mina Dulcan and D. Richard Martini, *Concise Guide to Child and Adolescent Psychiatry*, 2d ed. (Washington, D.C.: American Psychiatric Association Press, 1999), 259.

Chapter 7. MOOD-STABILIZING MEDICATIONS

1. Anastase Georgotas and Samuel Gershon, "Historical Perspectives and Current Highlights on Lithium Treatment in Manic-Depressive Illness," *Journal of Clinical Psychopharmacology* 1, no. 1 (1981): 27–31.

2. Many chemicals, including medications, consist of two parts called *ions*, one of which is positively charged (such as lithium or sodium) and the other negatively charged (such as chloride or carbonate). When the two parts exist together as a *compound*, the charges cancel each other out and the system is stable.

3. John F. J. Cade, "Lithium Salts in the Treatment of Psychotic Excitement," *Medical Journal of Australia* 36 (1949): 349–52.

4. Ibid., 350.

5. Ibid., 350–51.

6. Ronald R. Fieve, *Moodswing: The Third Revolution in Psychiatry* (New York: Bantam Books, 1975), 3.

7. M. Schou, N. Juel-Nielsen, E. Strömgren, and H. Voldby, "The Treatment

of Manic Psychoses by the Administration of Lithium Salts," *Journal of Neurology, Neurosurgery, and Psychiatry* 17 (1954): 250–60.

8. Paul Baalstrup and Morgans Schou, "Lithium as a Prophylactic Agent: Its Effect against Recurrent Depressions and Manic-Depressive Psychosis," *Archives of General Psychiatry* 16, no. 2 (1967): 162–72.

9. E. P. Worrall, J. P. Moody, and M. Peet, "Controlled Studies of the Acute Antidepressant Effects of Lithium," *British Journal of Psychiatry* 135 (1979): 255–62.

10. F. Rouillon and P. Gorwood, "The Use of Lithium to Augment Antidepressant Medication," *Journal of Clinical Psychiatry* 59, suppl. 5 (1998): 32–39.

11. Robert Kowatch and John Bucci, "Mood Stabilizers and Anticonvulsants," *Pediatric Clinics of North America* 45, no. 5 (1998): 1173–86.

12. To be more precise, the therapeutic index is the ratio of the largest dose producing no toxic symptoms to the smallest dose routinely producing the desired therapeutic effects.

13. We speak of a "therapeutic level" in discussing the effective range of lithium in the bloodstream for treatment, not a "normal level." Lithium is a trace element in the body, normally present in undetectable concentrations.

14. Morgans Schou, "Forty Years of Lithium Treatment," *Archives of General Psychiatry* 54 (1997): 9–13.

15. Ibid., 11.

16. Neal Ryan, Vinod Bhatara, and James Perel, "Mood Stabilizers in Children and Adolescents," *Journal of the American Academy of Child and Adolescent Psychiatry* 38, no. 5 (1999): 529–36.

17. Ibid.

18. G. Walter, B. Lyndon, and R. Kubb, "Lithium Augmentation of Venlafaxine in Adolescent Major Depression," *Australian and New Zealand Journal of Psychiatry* 32, no. 3 (1998): 457–59.

19. American Psychiatric Association, "Practice Guidelines for the Treatment of Bipolar Disorder," *American Journal of Psychiatry* 151, suppl. (1994): 7.

20. Frederick K. Goodwin and Kay Redfield Jamison, *Manic-Depressive Illness* (New York: Oxford University Press, 1990), 707.

21. See Charles Bowden and Susan McElroy, "History of the Development of Valproate for the Treatment of Bipolar Disorder," *Journal of Clinical Psychiatry* 56, suppl. 3 (1995): 3–5.

22. Charles L. Bowden, "Predictors of Response to Divalproex and Lithium," *Journal of Clinical Psychiatry* 56, suppl. 3 (1995): 25–29.

23. Susan McElroy, Paul Keck, Harrison Pope, and James Hudson, "Valproate in Psychiatric Disorders: Literature Review and Clinical Guidelines," *Journal of Clinical Psychiatry* 50, suppl. 3 (1989): 23–29.

24. American Psychiatric Association, "Practice Guidelines for the Treatment of Bipolar Disorder," 21. See also Alan Swann, Charles Bowden, David Morris, Joseph Calabrese, Frederick Petty, Joyce Small, Steven Dilsaver, and John Davis, "Depression during Mania: Treatment Response to Lithium or Divalproex," *Archives of General Psychiatry* 54 (1997): 37–42.

25. American Psychiatric Association, "Practice Guidelines for the Treatment of Bipolar Disorder," 10.

26. See Frederick Jacobson, "Low-Dose Valproate: A New Treatment for Cyclothymia, Mild Rapid-Cycling Disorders and Premenstrual Syndrome," *Journal of Clinical Psychiatry* 54, no. 6 (1993): 229–34. See also J. A. Delito, "The Effect of Valproate on Bipolar Spectrum Temperamental Disorders," *Journal of Clinical Psychiatry* 54, no. 8 (1993): 300–304.

27. Ryan, Bhatara, and Perel, "Mood Stabilizers in Children and Adolescents."

28. Gary Sachs, "Bipolar Mood Disorder: Practical Strategies for Acute and Maintenance Phase Treatment," *Journal of Clinical Psychopharmacology* 16, no. 2, suppl. 1 (1996): 32S–47S.

29. F. E. Dreifuss, D. H. Langer, K. A. Moline, and J. E. Maxwell, "Valproic Acid Hepatic Fatalities II: US Experience since 1984," *Neurology* 39, no. 2, pt. 1 (1989): 201–7.

30. Barbara Geller, "Valproate and Polycystic Ovaries," *Journal of the American Academy of Child and Adolescent Psychiatry* 537, no. 1 (1998): 9–10.

31. J. C. Ballenger and R. M. Post, "Carbamazepine in Manic-Depressive Illness: A New Treatment," *American Journal of Psychiatry* 37, no. 7 (1980): 782–90.

32. B. Lerer, M. Moore, E. Meyendorff, S. R. Cho, and S. Gershon, "Carbamazepine versus Lithium in Mania: A Double Blind Study," *Journal of Clinical Psychiatry* 48 (1987): 89–93.

33. Robert Post, Thomas Uhde, James Ballenger, and Kathleen Squillace, "Prophylactic Efficacy of Carbamazepine in Manic-Depressive Illness," *American Journal of Psychiatry* 140 (1983): 1602–4.

34. Joseph Woolston, "Case Study: Carbamazepine Treatment of Juvenile-Onset Bipolar Disorder," *Journal of the American Academy of Child and Adolescent Psychiatry*, 38, no. 3 (1999): 335–38.

35. Jonathan Sporn and Gary Sachs, "The Anticonvulsant Lamotrigine in Treatment Resistant Manic-Depressive Illness," *Journal of Clinical Psychopharmacology* 17 (1997): 185–89.

36. Joseph Calabrese, S. Hossein Fatemi, and Mark Woyshville, "Antidepressant Effects of Lamotrigine in Rapid Cycling Bipolar Disorder," *American Journal of Psychiatry* 153, no. 9 (1996): 1236.

37. Thomas Maltese, "Adjunctive Lamotrigine Treatment for Major Depression," *American Journal of Psychiatry* 156, no. 11 (1999): 1833.

38. Sporn and Sachs, "Anticonvulsant Lamotrigine in Treatment Resistant Manic-Depressive Illness."

39. Sean Stanton, Paul Keck, and Susan McElroy, "Treatment of Acute Mania with Gabapentin," *American Journal of Psychiatry* 154, no. 2 (1997): 287.

40. Charles Schaffer and Linda Schaffer, "Gabapentin in the Treatment of Bipolar Disorder," *American Journal of Psychiatry* 154, no. 2 (1997): 291.

41. Marshall Teitlebaum, "Oxycarbazepine in Bipolar Disorder," *Journal of the American Academy of Child and Adolescent Psychiatry* 40, no. 9 (2001): 993–94.

42. For a discussion of all these issues, see Magda Campbell and Jeanette Cueva,

"Psychopharmacology in Child and Adolescent Psychiatry: A Review of the Past Seven Years. Part II," *Journal of the American Academy of Child and Adolescent Psychiatry* 34, no. 10 (1995) 1262–72; and Ryan, Bhatara, and Perel, "Mood Stabilizers in Children and Adolescents."

Chapter 8. OTHER MEDICATIONS AND TREATMENTS

1. Magda Campbell, Judith Rapoport, and George Simpson, "Antipsychotics in Children and Adolescents," *Journal of the American Academy of Child and Adolescent Psychiatry* 38, no. 5 (1999): 537–45.

2. H. A. Scheier, "Risperidone for Young Children with Mood Disorders and Aggressive Behaviors," *Journal of Child and Adolescent Psychopharmacology* 8, no. 1 (1998): 49–59.

3. In a study of 11,555 patients treated with clozapine, 73 (or 0.91 percent) developed agranulocytosis (of whom 2 died of the infectious complications of the condition). See Jose Alvir, Jeffrey Lieberman, Allan Safferman, Jeffrey Schwimmer, and John Schaaf, "Clozapine-Induced Agranulocytosis: Incidence and Risk Factors in the United States," *New England Journal of Medicine* 329 (1993): 162–67.

4. K. Linde, G. Ramirez, C. D. Mulrow, A. Pauls, and W. Weidenhammer, "St. John's Wort for Depression—An Overview and Meta-analysis of Randomized Clinical Trials," *British Medical Journal* 3, no. 313 (1996): 253–58.

5. E. U. Vorbach, W. D. Hubner, and K. H. Arnoldt, "Effectiveness and Tolerance of the Hypericum Extract LI 160 in Comparison with Imipramine: Randomized Double-Blind Study with 135 Outpatients," *Journal of Geriatric Psychiatry and Neurology* 7, suppl. 1 (1994): S19–S23.

6. R. Bergman, J. Nuessner, and J. Demling, "Treatment of Mild to Moderate Depression: A Comparison between *Hypericum perforatum* and Amitriptyline," *Neurologie/Psychiatrie* 7 (1993) 235–40; summarized in Peter McWilliams, Mikael Nordfors, and Harold H. Bloomfield, *Hypericum and Depression* (Los Angeles: Prelude Press, 1996).

7. These studies compared effectiveness of hypericum preparations with doses of 75 mg of imipramine, a dose most psychiatrists would probably consider barely in the usually effective range, and 30 mg of amitriptyline, a dose that is definitely subtherapeutic for most patients.

8. Richard Shelton, Martin Keller, Alan Gelenberg, David Dunner, Robert Hirschfeld, Michael Thase, James Russel, R. Bruce Lydiard, Paul Crits-Christoph, Robert Gallop, Linda Todd, David Hellerstein, Paul Goodnick, Gabor Keitner, Stephen Stahl, and Uriel Halbreich, "Effectiveness of St. John's Wort in Major Depression: A Randomized Controlled Trial," *Journal of the American Medical Association* 285 (2001): 1978–86.

9. For a discussion of the plant origins and potent toxicity of several poisons, see Joel Hardman, Alfred Goodman Gilman, and Lee Limbird, *Goodman and Gilman's The Pharmacological Basis of Medical Therapeutics*, 9th ed. (New York: McGraw-Hill, Health Professions Division, 1996), 178–90 (strychnine and related compounds), 146–49 (amatoxins), and 149–54 (the belladonna alkaloids).

10. Andrew Stoll, Emanuel Severus, Marlene Freeman, Stephanie Rueter, Holly Zboyan, Eli Diamond, Kimberly Cress, and Lauren Marangell, "Omega 3 Fatty Acids in Bipolar Disorder: A Preliminary Double-Blind, Placebo-Controlled Trial," *Archives of General Psychiatry* 56, no. 5 (1999): 407–12.

11. Michael Alvear, "A True Fish Story," www.salon.com, Sept. 9, 1999.

12. Hiroyasu Iso, Kathryn Rexrode, Meir Stampfer, JoAnn Manson, Graham Cloditz, Frank Speizer, Charles Hennekens, and Walter Willett, "Intake of Fish and Omega-3 Fatty Acids and Risk of Stroke in Women," *Journal of the American Medical Association* 285, no. 3 (2001): 304–12.

13. Joseph Rey and Garry Walter, "Half a Century of ECT Use in Young People," *American Journal of Psychiatry* 154, no. 5 (1997): 595–602.

14. Garry Walter, Karryn Koster, and Joseph Rey, "Electroconvulsive Therapy in Adolescents: Experience, Knowledge, and Attitudes of Recipients," *Journal of the American Academy of Child and Adolescent Psychiatry* 38, no. 5 (1999): 594–99. For an excellent discussion of the history and current practice of ECT, see Max Fink, *Electroshock: Restoring the Mind* (New York: Oxford University Press, 1999).

15. Larry Squire, Pamela Slater, and Patricia Miller, "Retrograde Amnesia and Bilateral Electroconvulsive Therapy: Long Term Follow-Up," *Archives of General Psychiatry* 38 (1981): 89–95.

16. C. P. L. Freeman, D. Weeks, and R. E. Kendell, "ECT III: Patients Who Complain," *British Journal of Psychiatry* 137 (1980): 17–25.

17. Larry R. Squire and Pamela C. Slater, "Electroconvulsive Therapy and Complaints of Memory Dysfunction: A Prospective Three-Year Follow-Up Study," *British Journal of Psychiatry* 142 (1983): 1–8.

18. S. Kutcher and H. Robertson, "Electroconvulsive Therapy in Treatment-Resistant Bipolar Youth," *Journal of Child and Adolescent Psychopharmacology* 5 (1995): 167–75.

19. David Cohen, Olivier Taieb, Martine Flament, Nina Benoit, Sylvie Chevret, Maurice Corcos, Philippe Fossati, Philippe Jeammet, Jean-François Allilaire, and Michel Basquin, "Absence of Cognitive Impairment at Long-Term Follow-up in Adolescents Treated with ECT for Severe Mood Disorder," *American Journal of Psychiatry* 157, no. 3 (2000): 460–62.

20. I. Perkins and K. Tanaka, "The Controversy That Will Not Die Is the Treatment That Can and Does Save Lives: Electroconvulsive Therapy," *Adolescence* 14 (1979): 607–17.

21. Sukeb Mukherjee, Harold Sackeim, and David Schnur, "Electroconvulsive Therapy of Acute Manic Episodes: A Review of 50 Years' Experience," *American Journal of Psychiatry* 151 (1994): 169–76.

22. S. Mukherjee, H. Sackheim, and C. Lee, "Unilateral ECT in the Treatment of Manic Episodes," *Convulsive Therapy* 4 (1988): 74–80.

23. Frederick K. Goodwin and Kay Redfield Jamison, *Manic-Depressive Illness* (New York: Oxford University Press, 1990), 661.

24. Olivier Taieb, David Cohen, Philippe Mezet, and Martine Flament, "Ado-

lescents' Experiences with ECT," *Journal of the American Academy of Child and Adolescent Psychiatry* 39, no. 8 (2000): 934–44.

25. See Mark S. George, Eric Wasserman, and Robert Post, "Transcranial Magnetic Stimulation: A Neuropsychiatric Tool for the 21st Century," *Journal of Neuropsychiatry and Clinical Neurosciences* 8 (1996): 373–82.

26. Mark George, Eric Wasserman, Tim Kimbrell, John Little, Wendol Williams, Aimee Danielson, Benjamin Greenberg, Mark Hallett, and Robert Post, "Mood Improvement Following Daily Left Prefrontal Repetitive Transcranial Magnetic Stimulation in Patients with Depression: A Placebo-Controlled Crossover Trial," *American Journal of Psychiatry* 154 (1997): 1752–56.

27. Mark George, Ziad Nahas, Monica Molloy, Andrew Speer, Nicholas Oliver, Xing-Bao Li, George Arana, S. Craig Risch, and James Ballenger, "A Controlled Trial of Daily Left Prefrontal Cortex TMS for Treating Depression," *Biological Psychiatry* 48 (2000): 962–70.

28. A. Pascual-Leone, B. Rubio, F. Pallardo, and M. D. Catala, "Beneficial Effect of Rapid-Rate Transcranial Magnetic Stimulation of the Left Dorsolateral Prefrontal Cortex in Drug-Resistant Depression," *Lancet* 348 (1996): 233–37; and Charles Epstein, Gary Figiel, William McDonald, Jody Amazon-Leece, and Linda Figiel, "Rapid Rate Transcranial Magnetic Stimulation in Young and Middle-Aged Refractory Depressed Patients," *Psychiatric Annals* 28 (1998): 36–39.

29. A. John Rush, Mark George, Harold Sackeim, Lauren Marangell, Mustafa Husain, Cole Giller, Ziad Nahas, Stephen Haines, Richard Simpson, and Robert Goodman, "Vagus Nerve Stimulation (VNS) for Treatment-Resistant Depression: A Multi-center Study," *Biological Psychiatry* 47, no. 4 (2000) 276–86.

Chapter 9. COUNSELING AND PSYCHOTHERAPY

1. A. Wood, R. Harrington, and A. Moore, "A Controlled Trial of Brief Cognitive-Behavioral Intervention in Adolescent Patients with Depressive Disorders," *Journal of Child Psychology and Psychiatry* 37 (1996): 737–46.

2. Boris Birmaher, David Brent, David Kolko, Marianne Baugher, Jeffrey Bridge, Diane Holder, Satish Iyengar, and Rosa Ulloa, "Clinical Outcome after Short-Term Psychotherapy for Adolescents with Major Depressive Disorder," *Archives of General Psychiatry* 57 (2000): 29–36.

3. Dinah Jayson, "Which Depressed Patients Respond to Cognitive-Behavioral Treatment?" *Journal of the American Academy of Child and Adolescent Psychiatry* 37, no. 1 (1998): 35–39.

4. Many, but not all, experts agree that the superiority of combination treatment is supported by research. See Jacqueline Persons, Michael Thase, and Paul Crits-Christoph, "The Role of Psychotherapy in the Treatment of Depression: A Review of Two Practice Guidelines," *Archives of General Psychiatry* 53 (1996): 283–90.

5. Jerome Frank, *Persuasion and Healing: A Comparative Study of Psychotherapy*, rev. ed. (New York: Schocken Books, 1974), xvi.

6. The standard work on cognitive-behavioral therapy is Aaron Beck, A. John

Rush, Brian Shaw, and Gary Emery, *Cognitive Therapy of Depression* (New York: Guilford Press, 1979).

7. The area of comparison studies of cognitive-behavioral psychotherapy and medication in the treatment of depression can be accurately described as a hornet's nest of controversy. It's not difficult to find a study to support any possible view: superiority of medication over psychotherapy, superiority of psychotherapy over medication, and equal efficacy for both. For a nicely designed and well-executed study that found that cognitive therapy was as helpful as imipramine for 107 patients with major depressive disorder, see Steven Hollon, Robert DeRubeis, Mark Evans, Marlin Wiemer, Michael Garvey, William Grove, and Vincente Tuason, "Cognitive Therapy and Pharmacotherapy for Depression, Singly and in Combination," *Archives of General Psychiatry* 49 (1992): 774–81. For readers who would like to jump into the hornet's nest, I suggest Persons, Thase, and Crits-Christoph, "The Role of Psychotherapy in the Treatment of Depression," and the four (yes, four) accompanying rebuttal/commentary articles in the same issue of *Archives of General Psychiatry*.

8. Beck et al., *Cognitive Therapy of Depression*, 11.

9. Laura Mufson, Myra Weissman, Donna Morceau, and Robin Garfinkle, "Efficacy of Interpersonal Psychotherapy for Depressed Adolescents," *Archives of General Psychiatry* 56 (1999): 573–79.

Chapter 10. ATTENTION-DEFICIT/HYPERACTIVITY DISORDER

1. George Still, "Some Abnormal Psychical Conditions in Childhood," *Lancet* 1 (1902): 1008–12.

2. Laurence Greenhill, Jeffrey Halperin, and Howard Abikoff, "Stimulant Medications," *Journal of the American Academy of Child and Adolescent Psychiatry* 38, no. 5 (1999): 503–12.

3. Arthur Robin, "Attention-Deficit/Hyperactivity Disorder in Adolescents," *Journal of the American Academy of Child and Adolescent Psychiatry* 45, no. 5 (1999): 1027–38.

4. Thomas Spencer, Joseph Biederman, and Timothy Wilens, "Attention-Deficit/Hyperactivity Disorder and Co-morbidity," *Pediatric Clinics of North America* 46, no. 5 (1999): 915–27.

5. J. Biederman, S. Faraone, E. Mick. J. Wozniac, L. Chen, C. Ouellette, A. Marrs, J. Garcia, D. Mennin, and E. Lelon, "Attention-Deficit Hyperactivity Disorder and Juvenile Mania: An Overlooked Comorbidity?" *Journal of the American Academy of Child and Adolescent Psychiatry* 35, no. 8 (1996): 997–1008.

6. Stephen Faraone, Joseph Biederman, Douglas Mennin, Janet Wozniak, and Thomas Spencer, "Attention-Deficit/Hyperactivity Disorder with Bipolar Disorder: A Familial Subtype?" *Journal of the American Academy of Child and Adolescent Psychiatry* 36, no. 10 (1997): 1378–87.

7. M. Strober, M. DeAntonio, S. Schmidt-Lackner, R. Freeman, C. Lampert, and J. Diamond, "Early Childhood Attention-Deficit/Hyperactivity Disorder Pre-

dicts Poorer Response to Acute Lithium Therapy in Adolescent Mania," *Journal of Affective Disorders* 51, no. 11 (1998): 145–51.

8. J. Biederman and T. Spencer, "Non-stimulant Treatment for ADHD," *European Child and Adolescent Psychiatry* 9, suppl. 1 (2000): 151–59.

Chapter II. ALCOHOL AND DRUG ABUSE

1. L. Johnston, P. O'Malley, J. Bachman, *Monitoring the Future: National Results on Adolescent Drug Abuse: Overview of Key Findings* (Bethesda, Md.: National Institute on Drug Abuse, 2001), 6.

2. Markus Henriksson, Hillevi Aro, Mauri Marttunnen, Martti Heikkinen, Erkki Isometsä, Kimmo Kuoppasalmi, and Jouko Lönnqvist, "Mental Disorders and Comorbidity in Suicide, *American Journal of Psychiatry* 150 (1993): 935–40.

3. Marjorie Hogan, "Diagnosis and Treatment of Teen Drug Use," *Medical Clinics of North America* 84, no. 4 (2000): 927–66.

4. Sandra Morrison, Peter Rogers, and Mark Thomas, "Alcohol and Adolescents," *Pediatric Clinics of North America* 42, no. 2 (1995): 371–87.

5. Andrew Johns, "Psychiatric Effects of Cannabis," *British Journal of Psychiatry* 178 (2001): 116–22.

6. Thomas Crowley, Marilyn Macdonald, Elizabeth Whitmore, and Susan Mikulich, "Cannabis Dependence, Withdrawal and Reinforcing Effects among Adolescents with Conduct Symptoms and Substance Abuse Disorders," *Drug and Alcohol Dependence* 50 (1998): 27–37.

7. Asbjørg Chrisopherson, "Amphetamine Designer Drugs—An Overview and Epidemiology," *Toxicology Letters* 112 (2000): 127–31.

8. For an excellent summary of MDMA's short-term and long-term effects on the brain, see Michael John Morgan, "Ecstasy (MDMA): A Review of Its Possible Persistent Psychological Effects" *Psychopharmacology* 152 (2000): 230–48.

9. Oscar Bukstein and the Work Group on Quality Issues of the American Academy of Child and Adolescent Psychiatry, "Practice Parameters for the Assessment and Treatment of Children and Adolescents with Substance Abuse Disorders," *Journal of the American Academy of Child and Adolescent Psychiatry* 36, no. 10S (1997): 140S–156S.

10. Timothy Wilens, Joseph Biederman, Ana Abrantes, and Thomas Spencer, "Clinical Characteristics of Psychiatrically Referred Adolescent Outpatients with Substance Abuse Disorder," *Journal of the American Academy of Child and Adolescent Psychiatry* 36, no. 7 (1997): 941–47.

11. Judith Brook, Patricia Cohen, and David Brook, "Longitudinal Study of Co-occurring Psychiatric Disorders and Substance Use," *Journal of the American Academy of Child and Adolescent Psychiatry* 37, no. 3 (1998): 322–30.

12. Michael Lyvers, "'Loss of Control' in Alcoholism and Drug Addiction: A Neuroscientific Interpretation," *Experimental and Clinical Psychopharmacology* 8, no. 2 (2000): 225–49.

13. Paul Bergman, Maurice Smith, and Norman Hoffman, "Adolescent Treat-

ment, Implications for Assessment, Practice Guidelines and Outcome Management," *Pediatric Clinics of North America* 42, no. 2 (1995): 453–72.

Chapter 12. EATING DISORDERS

1. The complete texts of all three historical accounts can be found in Arnold Anderson, *Practical Comprehensive Treatment of Anorexia and Bulimia* (Baltimore: Johns Hopkins University Press, 1985), 10–29.

2. Richard Kreipe and Susan Birndorf, "Eating Disorders in Adolescents," *Medical Clinics of North America* 84, no. 4 (2000): 1027–49.

3. Peter Lewinsohn, Ruth Striegel-Moore, and John Seeley, "Epidemiology and Natural Course of Eating Disorders in Young Women from Adolescence to Young Adulthood," *Journal of the American Academy of Child and Adolescent Psychiatry* 39, no. 10 (2000): 1284–92.

4. T. Zaider, J. Johnson, and S. Cockell, "Psychiatric Comorbidity Associated with Eating Disorder Symptomatology among Adolescents in the Community," *International Journal of Eating Disorders* 28, no. 1 (2000): 58–67.

5. Tracey Wade, Cynthia Bulik, Michael Neale, and Kenneth Kendler, "Anorexia Nervosa and Major Depression: Shared Genetic and Environmental Risk Factors," *American Journal of Psychiatry* 157, no. 3 (2000): 469–71.

6. A. Raffi, M. Rondini, S. Grandi, and G. Fava, "Life Events and Prodromal Symptoms in Bulimia Nervosa," *Psychological Medicine* 30, no. 3 (2000): 727–31.

7. David Jimerson, Barbara Wolfe, Andrew Brotman, and Eran Metzger, "Medications in the Treatment of Eating Disorders," *Psychiatric Clinics of North America* 19, no. 4 (1996): 739–54.

8. Walter Kaye, Kelly Gendell, and Michael Strober, "Serotonin Neuronal Function and Selective Serotonin Reuptake Inhibitor Treatment in Anorexia and Bulimia Nervosa," *Biological Psychiatry* 44 (1998): 825–38.

Chapter 13. "CUTTING" AND OTHER SELF-HARMING BEHAVIORS

1. Paul R. McHugh and Phillip R. Slavney, *The Perspectives of Psychiatry* (Baltimore: Johns Hopkins University Press, 1999), 151.

2. Jennifer Egan, "The Thin Red Line," *New York Times Magazine*, July 27, 1997.

3. Armando Favazza, "The Coming of Age of Self-Mutilation," *Journal of Nervous and Mental Disease* 186, no. 5 (1998): 259–68.

4. Caron Zlotnick, Jill Mattia, and Mark Zimmerman, "Clinical Correlates of Self-Mutilation in a Sample of General Psychiatric Patients," *Journal of Nervous and Mental Diseases* 187, no. 5 (1999): 296–301.

5. Favazza, "Coming of Age of Self-Mutilation."

6. See Egan, "Thin Red Line"; and Marilee Strong, *A Bright Red Scream: Self-Mutilation and the Language of Pain* (New York: Penguin Books, 1999).

7. See Armando Favazza, *Bodies under Siege: Self-Mutilation and Body Modification in Culture and Psychiatry*, 2d ed. (Baltimore: Johns Hopkins University Press, 1996), 241.

8. Marsha Linehan, *Cognitive-Behavioral Therapy of the Borderline Personality Disorder* (New York: Guilford Press, 1993).

9. Alan Frances, "Introduction to Section on Self-Mutilation," *Journal of Personality Disorders* 1 (1987): 316.

10. For a review of all the statistics cited in this section, see David Clark, "Suicidal Behavior in Childhood and Adolescence: Recent Studies and Clinical Implications," *Psychiatric Annals* 23, no. 5 (1993): 271–83; and Iris Borowski, Marjorie Ireland, and Michael Resnick, "Adolescent Suicide Attempts: Risks and Protectors," *Pediatrics* 107, no. 3 (2001): 485–93.

11. David Shaffer, Madelyn Gould, Prudence Fisher, Paul Trautman, Donna Moreau, Marjorie Kleinman, and Michael Flory, "Psychiatric Diagnosis in Child and Adolescent Suicide," *Archives of General Psychiatry* 53, no. 4 (1996): 339–48.

12. Iris Borowski, Marjorie Ireland, and Michael Resnick, "Adolescent Suicide Attempts: Risks and Protectors," *Pediatrics* 107, no. 3 (2001): 485–93.

13. Centers for Disease Control, "Effectiveness in Disease and Injury Prevention: Adolescent Suicide and Suicide Attempts—Santa Fe County, New Mexico, January 1985–May 1990," *Morbidity and Mortality Weekly Report* 40, no. 20 (1990): 329–31.

14. D. Brent, J. Perper, C. Allman, G. Moritz, M. Wartella, and J. Zelenak, "The Presence and Accessibility of Firearms in the Homes of Adolescent Suicides: A Case Control Study," *Journal of the American Medical Association* 266, no. 21 (1991): 2989–95.

15. David Schaffer and Leslie Craft, "Methods of Adolescent Suicide Prevention," *Journal of Clinical Psychiatry* 60, suppl. 2 (1999): 70–74.

Chapter 14. THE GENETICS OF MOOD DISORDERS

1. Emil Kraepelin, *Manic-Depressive Insanity and Paranoia*, trans. R. M. Barclay, ed. G. M. Robertson (Edinburgh: E. & S. Livingstone, 1921; reprinted New York: Arno Press, 1976), 165 (in reprint edition).

2. For a more detailed account, which includes references to the original articles, see Eliot Marshall, "Manic Depression: Highs and Lows on the Research Roller Coaster," *Science* 264 (1994): 1693–95.

3. An overview of this work is provided in Melvin McGinnis, "Recent Advances in the Genetics of Bipolar Disorder," *Psychiatric Annals* 27 (1997): 482–88.

4. See Elliot S. Gershon, "Genetics," in *Manic-Depressive Illness*, Frederick K. Goodwin and Kay Redfield Jamison (New York: Oxford University Press, 1990), 373–401.

5. For a very readable overview of some of these issues, see Doris Teichler Zallen, *Does It Run in the Family? A Consumer's Guide to DNA Testing for Genetic Disorders* (New Brunswick, N.J.: Rutgers University Press, 1997).

Chapter 15. STRATEGIES FOR SUCCESSFUL TREATMENT

1. Emil Kraepelin, *Manic-Depressive Insanity and Paranoia*, trans. R. M. Barclay, ed. G. M. Robertson (Edinburgh: E. & S. Livingstone, 1921; reprinted New York: Arno Press, 1976), pp. 179–181 (in reprint edition).

2. Ian M. Goodyer, "The Influence of Recent Life Events on the Onset and Outcome of Major Depression in Young People," in *Depressive Disorders in Children and Adolescents: Epidemiology, Risk Factors, and Treatment*, ed. Cecilia Ahmoi Essau and Franz Petermann (Northvale, N.J.: Jason Aronson, 1999), 241.

3. For a complete discussion of these animal models of the kindling phenomenon, see Robert Post, "Transduction of Psychosocial Stress into the Neurobiology of Recurrent Affective Disorder," *American Journal of Psychiatry* 149 (1992): 999–1010.

4. Constance Hammen and Michael Gitlin, "Stress Reactivity in Bipolar Patients and Its Relation to Prior History of Disorder," *American Journal of Psychiatry* 154 (1997): 856–57.

5. Depression Guideline Panel, *Depression in Primary Care*, vol. 1, *Treatment of Major Depression: Clinical Practice Guidelines* (Rockville, Md.: U.S. Department of Health and Human Services, Public Health Service, Agency for Health Care Policy and Research, 1993).

6. George McGovern, *Terry: My Daughter's Life-and-Death Struggle with Alcoholism* (New York: Villard Books, 1996), 187.

7. See Peter Lewinsohn, Paul Rohde, John Seeley, Daniel Klein, and Ian Gotlib, "Natural Course of Adolescent Major Depressive Disorder in a Community Sample: Predictors of Recurrence in Young Adults," *American Journal of Psychiatry* 157, no. 10 (2000): 1584–91; and Mark Sanford, Peter Szatmari, Miriam Spinner, Heather Munroe-Blum, Ellen Jamison, Christine Walsh, and Debbie Jones, "Predicting the One-Year Course of Adolescent Major Depression," *Journal of the American Academy of Child and Adolescent Psychiatry* 34, no. 12 (1994): 1618–28.

Chapter 16. THE ROLE OF THE FAMILY

1. Stephen Strakowski, Susan McElroy, Paul Keck, and Scott West, "Suicidality among Patients with Mixed and Manic Bipolar Disorder," *American Journal of Psychiatry* 153 (1996): 674–76.

Chapter 17. PLANNING FOR EMERGENCIES

1. See, for example, J. E. Bailey, A. L. Kellerman, G. W. Somes, J. G. Banton, F. P. Rivara, and N. P. Rushforth, "Risk Factors for Violent Death of Women in the Home," *Archives of Internal Medicine* 157 (1997): 777–82.

Index

brain imaging, 260
buproprion, 97, 169

Cade, John F. J., 104–5
carbamazepine: side effects, 118–19; therapeutic profile, 117–18
Carpenter, Karen, 187
Catapres, 169
Celexa, 96
chlordiazepoxide, 129
chlorpromazine, 125
citalopram, 96
clomipramine, 91
clonazepam, 129
clonidine, 169
clorazepate, 129
clozapine, 127, 128
Clozaril, 127
cocaine abuse, 179, 181, 231
Cognex, 169
commitment (for involuntary treatment), 243–46
conduct disorder, 61, 122
counseling, 224. *See also* psychotherapy
cyclothymic disorder, 52–53, 54, 55

DBT (dialectical-behavioral therapy), 198
delusions, 22–23, 36, 39–40, 69, 124
demoralization, 28–30
denial, 175
Depakene. *See* valproate
Depakote. *See* valproate
depression: classification of, 55–59; definition of, 7–8, 13; diagnosis of, 2; prevalence of, xi, 27–28, 41; switch into bipolar disorder, 55; undertreatment of, xii
depressive equivalent, 21
desipramine, 91
developmental foreclosure, 27
developmental theory: of Erik Erikson, 24–27; of G. Stanley Hall, 23–24; of James Marcia, 27

dextroamphetamine, 167
diabetes insipidus, 111
diagnosis: importance of, 218–21; the diagnostic process in psychiatry, 3, 33–35
Diagnostic and Statistical Manual of Mental Disorders. See DSM
dialectical-behavioral therapy (DBT), 198
diazepam, 129
diurnal variation of mood, 16
donepezil, 170
dopamine, 85, 124–25
double-blind clinical studies, 93–94
double depression, 45
doxepin, 91
DRADA (Depressive and Related Affective Disorders Association), 264
DSM (*Diagnostic and Statistical Manual of Mental Disorders*): classification axes, 64–67; history of, 62–63; mood disorders in, 70
dual diagnosis, 182–84
dysphoria, 35
dysthymic disorder: *vs.* major depression, 46; symptoms of, 43–46

eating disorders: anorexia nervosa, 188–89; binge-eating disorder, 190; bulimia nervosa, 189–90; classification of, 187–88; relationship to mood disorders, 193–94; social factors as causes of, 191–92
"ecstasy" (MDMA), 177–80
ECT. *See* electroconvulsive therapy
Effexor, 97
"Eight Stages of Man" (Erickson), 24–25
Elavil. *See* amitriptyline
Eldepryl, 98
electroconvulsive therapy (ECT): description of, 136–38; development of, 134–36; for mania, 140; mechanism of action, 139; prescription for

adolescents, 139–40; side effects, 137–39
EPS (extrapyramidal symptoms), 128
Erikson, Eric, 24–27

family therapy, 154–55
fatty acids, 113, 131–34
FDA (Food and Drug Administration), 76–78
Fieve, Ronald, 106
fish oil, 131–33
fluoxetine, ix, 85, 96
fluphenazine, 126
fluvoxamine, 96
Frank, Jerome, 28–29, 150
Freud, Anna, 29, 175
Freud, Sigmund, 175

GABA (gamma-aminobutyric acid), 114
gabapentin, 121
Gabatril, 122
GAF scale, 66–67
genetics, 205–13, 260–61
Geodon, 127
Global Assessment of Functioning (GAF) scale, 66–67
Goethe, Johann Wolfgang, 13
G proteins, 86–87
group therapy, 156–57
guanfacine, 169

Haldol, 126
half-life of pharmaceuticals, 108
Hall, G. Stanley, 23
hallucinations, 19, 22–23, 36, 69, 124
haloperidol, 126
Huntington's disease, 209
Hypericum perforatum, 129–31
hypomania, 48, 51
hypothyroidism, 112

identity diffusion, 26
imipramine, 83, 91, 130
interpersonal psychotherapy, 153–54

involuntary commitment, 243–46
iproniazide, 83
irritability, 8–9, 13, 40, 48, 122, 168

James, William, 7

kindling theory of mood disorders, 230–31
Kinsey, Alfred, 31
Klonapin, 129
Kraepelin, Emil, 57, 230
Kuhn, Roland, 83, 91

Lamictal. See lamotrigine
lamotrigine: side effects, 120–21; therapeutic profile, 119–20
Librium, 129
Linehan, Marcia, 198
lithium: description, 103–4; mechanism of action, 86–87; side effects, 110–13; therapeutic profile, 107–9
lorazepam, 129
loxapine, 126
Loxitane, 126
Ludiomil, 91
Luvox, 96

major depressive disorder: course of illness, 42; symptoms of, 35–41
managed care, 255
mania: ECT for, 140; symptoms of, 46–47. See also bipolar disorder
manic-depression, 57. See also bipolar disorder
MAOIs (monoamine oxidase inhibitors), 98–100
maprotiline, 91
marijuana abuse, 176–77, 234–35; treatment issues, 182–84
"masked depression," 21
McGovern, Senator George, 235, 264
McHugh, Paul R., 195
MDMA ("ecstasy"), 177–80
Meduna, Joseph Ladislas von, 134